**SHW**

## Client Endorsements

*Since beginning Pilates with Karena, my osteoporosis has been downgraded to osteopoenia (low bone density, but not as severe as osteoporosis), and that was before I added medication to my treatment plan. I also have learned how to do everything I love (such as dancing) without risk of fracture. I don't want to live in fear of another fracture, and with the safe movement guidelines I have learned, I don't have to.*

—Phyllis Elias

*When I fractured my wrist, I found that I had osteoporosis. I began Pilates to increase my bone density, but it has resulted in much more than that. I am more flexible, stronger, and I have a lot more energy. It has also helped greatly with depression. I feel a greatly increased sense of well-being.*

—Shirley Potter

*With the help of Pilates exercises that have been modified to be safe for osteoporosis, my diagnosis of osteoporosis has been reduced to osteopoenia, which is a significant improvement. I have also improved my posture, balance, strength, flexibility, and stamina, which affords me a greater feeling of security when walking, climbing stairs, or just going through my everyday routine.*

—Betty Gildersleeve, R.N.

*After bodybuilding for many years I herniated two discs in my back. Being able to do nothing at all was not working for me. I discovered Pilates, and not only is my back stronger, but my entire body is enjoying the benefits. Pilates has made an enormous difference in my life.*

—Debbie Fecteau

*Pilates has strengthened my body both physically and mentally. Last year after I had a hysterectomy, I was able to return to exercise within a 10-day period. I felt so strong after my surgery and was able to deal with the emotional aspect of it all. Pilates seems to keep my balance between motherhood, raising a family, and owning my own business; it has helped me tremendously. Karena's program is one of the best, and she explains all positions to the point where a beginner can start right away and feel the results immediately.*

—Lisa Glogow

# Osteo Pilates

## INCREASE BONE DENSITY
## REDUCE FRACTURE RISK
## LOOK AND FEEL GREAT!

*By*

# KARENA THEK LINEBACK

NEW PAGE BOOKS
A division of The Career Press, Inc.
Franklin Lakes, NJ

OSTEOPILATES
EDITED BY CLAYTON W. LEADBETTER
TYPESET BY EILEEN DOW MUNSON
Cover design by Lu Rossman/Digi Dog Design
Printed in the U.S.A. by Book-mart Press

To order this title, please call toll-free 1-800-CAREER-1 (NJ and Canada: 201-848-0310) to order using VISA or MasterCard, or for further information on books from Career Press.

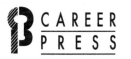 

The Career Press, Inc., 3 Tice Road, PO Box 687,
Franklin Lakes, NJ 07417
**www.careerpress.com**
**www.newpagebooks.com**

**Library of Congress Cataloging-in-Publication Data**

Lineback, Karena Thek.
    Osteopilates / by Karena Thek Lineback.
        p. cm.
    Includes index.
    ISBN 1-56414-687-1 (pbk.)
        1. Osteoporosis—Prevention. 2. Osteoporosis—Exercise therapy. 3. Pilates method. I. Title.

RC931.O73L554 2003
616.7'16--dc21

                                            2003042155

To my husband:
    Without you, this book
would have been truly impossible.

To my son:
    Thank you for giving up
    computer games so
    I could write this book.

    I love you both.

To my parents:
    Your unwavering love
    and support is cherished.

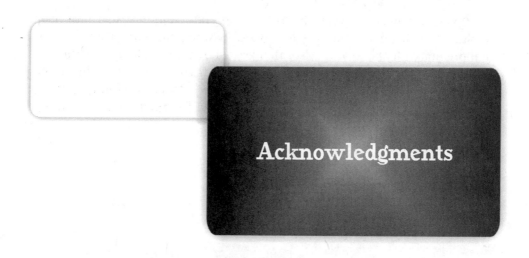

# Acknowledgments

I need to first acknowledge all of the work that my husband—my first editor—put into this book. He took what appeared to be mostly stream-of-consciousness writing and began to mold it into a much more legible form. Thanks go out to Clayton Leadbetter, my editor at Career Press, who took that legible form and made it into a work of art. Briana Rosen, thank you not only for the beautiful book cover, but for your encouragement. New England Publishing Associates and, especially, Elizabeth Frost-Knappmann deserve so much of the credit for not only accepting my proposal but for being excited about *OsteoPilates* and pitching it to publishers. Special thanks to Dennis Mecham of Salt Lake City, Utah for his artistic vision that shines through in his photography, which is thoroughly apparent throughout this book. Georgio Simeon, thank you for seeing that this book could be beneficial to so many thousands of people and taking the time to publicize it and to help me learn about the world of book marketing.

A million thanks to the world's best marketing team, my parents—Richard and Regina Thek. If the soda companies had these two working for them, there would no longer be water coming out of your kitchen faucet. Thanks to all my family and friends for believing in me and encouraging me through the somewhat daunting process of putting a book together. There's nothing more encouraging than having a friend backflip out of her chair with happiness when she is sharing your good news (Chrissy Schreibstein, Pammy Sue Vanderway, and Courtney B. Norris). I also have to mention Annie Cook, who was the first to say, "Write it, it's a great idea!" Special thanks go out to my son, who is as happy for me when I publish a book as he is when I bowl a strike—you keep things in better perspective than anyone I know.

Special thanks to all my clients for their endorsements that have been included in this book and for their week-by-week support of all that was happening with this book. Also, thanks to Dr. Parviz Galdjie of the Osteoporosis Institute in Santa Clarita, California and Dr. Christiane Northrup, author of *Women's Bodies, Women's Wisdom* (Bantam 1998) and *The Wisdom of Menopause* (Bantam 2001) for their support and endorsements of *OsteoPilates*.

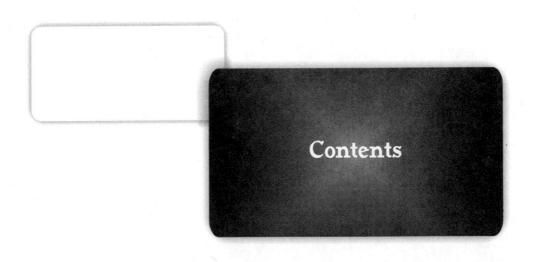

# Contents

Part Two:
OsteoPilates Exercises
101

# Foreword
by
Parviz Galdjie,
M.D., F.I.C.S.

Osteoporosis is moving, and rightfully so, to the forefront of women's health issues. It is so unfortunate that such a preventable and now treatable condition is allowed, and so sadly, to affect and alter the quality of life, as well as life itself, in so many millions of women. So it was a great pleasure for me to review this very nicely written and illustrated book. *OsteoPilates* provides a wide spectrum of well-needed information and, even more importantly, instructions for specific Pilates exercises to assist the general public—in particular, women—to become actively involved in their own care, thus slowing down and even hopefully reversing some of the bone mass losses which already may have occurred.

Following instructions recommended in this book (diet, calcium and other nutritional supplements, appropriate bone densitometry testing, and of course, the main emphasis of the book—Pilates exercises) will save thousands of women from the agony of fracture and deformities, which would be inevitable if this silent disease is ignored.

I recommend this book strongly. I believe a copy should be present in every family and it should be read by all members of the family—particularly the women of all ages.

—Parviz Galdjie, M.D., F.I.C.S.
**Osteoporosis Institute**
23838 Valencia Blvd.
Suite #150
Santa Clarita, CA 91355
661-253-0142

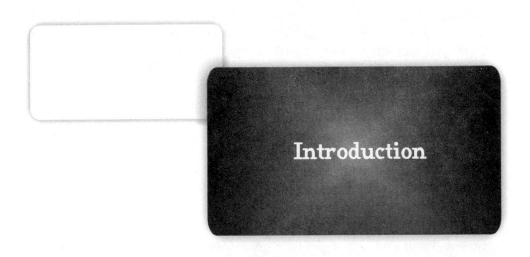

# Introduction

This book had to be written. It was one of those things in a person's life for which there really doesn't appear to be an option. The lack of information on living and exercising safely with osteoporosis is appalling. These guidelines are probably our healthcare system's best kept secret. I truly believe that once the knowledge in this book becomes commonplace, when bone density scans become routine and when preventative measures are taken for people who are at high risk, osteoporosis will become a disease of the past. Many health professionals with whom I have spoken call osteoporosis "the most easily preventable disease." But it's *not* being prevented. The information was not available. Too many patients are exercising to increase their bone density in hopes of combating osteoporosis, but are, in fact, increasing their fracture risk through dangerous movement patterns.

Sadly, I've never spoken to anyone with osteoporosis who was familiar with the safe movement guidelines that were given to me during my very first exercise certification class. Because they weren't a mystery to me, someone without osteoporosis, I couldn't understand why they were such a mystery to the people who could be seriously injured or even crippled by violating these safe movement guidelines. So I went online and searched for the information. I went to bookstores. I couldn't find anything anywhere (except in my professional books, and most people with osteoporosis aren't reading those) about exercising and living safely with osteoporosis.

There is plenty of information available about preventing a fall, but in my experience, that isn't where a good portion of fractures happen. I had a young client (early 40s) with osteopoenia who fractured her spine at the local gym doing abdominal crunches. Can you imagine anything more discouraging? She knew she had low bone density and she was trying to improve it, only to end up with a fracture. If it had been me, I probably would have quit exercising, thinking that no matter what I did I was doomed to break my bones. These fractures that occur during an exercise situation leave most people thinking that they have only strained their back or "overdid" an exercise or two when, in reality, they are actually creating a serious injury. In some cases, many tiny fractures can accumulate before a woman sees her doctor about the increasing pain in her back. The more that these tiny fractures accumulate, the more the deformity of the spine increases— and so does that person's dependence on others. So you see, this book *had* to be written.

I encourage you to read on and learn everything there is to know about osteoporosis. As my husband always says, "forewarned is forearmed." Not only will you find safe movement guidelines and an entire exercise program designed to be safe for osteoporosis within this book, but you will also find all the nuts and bolts of osteoporosis. You'll learn what causes osteoporosis (perhaps there is a habit that you have that is decreasing your bone density even now), how menopause affects a woman's bone density, what dietary habits will help to improve bone density, and which medications are available to you for increasing bone density.

Good luck on your journey for improving your health. The mere fact that you have purchased this book shows that you are the type of person who is holding the reins and not being led around by the horse (no matter how big). I have had many clients improve their bone density, and you can too. You can do it!

# Part One

## The Facts About Osteoporosis and Bone Density

## Chapter 1

### One in Two Women (and Other Osteoporosis Secrets)

▶ Fifty percent of women and 12 percent of men will suffer an osteoporosis–related break after reaching the age of 50.

▶ The expense for hospitals and nursing homes nationwide, for osteoporosis and associated fractures, is $17 billion each year, or $47 million each day.

▶ There are more than one million osteoporosis fractures each year, including:

- 300,000 hip fractures.

- 700,000 spinal fractures.

- 250,000 wrist fractures.

- 300,000 fractures in additional locations.

▶ The likelihood of a woman suffering a hip fracture is more than that of breast and ovarian cancer combined.

## What Happens After a Hip Fracture?

▶ Of hip fracture patients older than 50, approximately one in four die in the year following the break. Twice as many men than women will die after a hip fracture.

▶ Almost 25 percent of people who fracture their hip must relinquish their homes for long-term care or rehabilitation facilities.

# A Few Thin Bones—How Bad Could It Be?

Two types of osteoporotic clients walk through my door. The first group understands the fracture risk inherent in osteoporosis and wants to learn all there is to know about how to prevent a broken bone. I have to be honest and say that I have only met one person who fits that bill. The second, more common group reads the statistics but still isn't sold on the fact that they could break a bone due to osteoporosis—even if they already have! Individuals in the second group tell me, "Well, I just have a little bit of osteoporosis," or "I don't have osteoporosis very badly." True, there are degrees of bone loss, but if you have been *diagnosed* with osteoporosis, then your bone loss is already medically labeled as "severe and established." If you still aren't sold, or if you are young and need convincing to swallow a few more calcium tablets, then the following—and very real—scenario is for you. And by the way, most people do not believe that they will ever suffer a fracture. They are sure they are not part of the 50 percent of women who will suffer an osteoporosis fracture during their life. Please read on...

It is another beautiful morning and you are getting ready to go grocery shopping with a friend. Up until a few months ago, grocery shopping was an annoying task that you fit in between all of your other errands for the day. However, recently it has become a much bigger outing, since you can no longer drive. Your last visit to the doctor revealed exactly what you were afraid of: another fracture in your spine. You were hoping that it was just some nagging back pain, but since this is your third vertebral fracture, you had pretty much guessed it wasn't just muscle pain. The pain in your back makes driving very difficult, so your doctor has issued a temporary handicapped parking tag while you wait for the permanent tag to come in. Once at the store you wait for your friend to help you out of the car. You feel embarrassed to cling to her arm as you walk, but you know you just couldn't bear one more fracture, so you give in to help. From the grocery store you head to the mall. You catch a glimpse of yourself in the mirror-lined entryway. The vertebral fractures have left you with a dowager's hump and a potbelly. You remember when you were a little girl and your mother used to always say, "Stand up straight!" You'd yank your shoulders back and suck your stomach in. You wish it were that easy now. No amount of yanking or sucking can change the deformities that osteoporosis can create. Now in the woman's section of a large department store, you head for the plus size rack. You're not overweight and were always a size 10 or 12, but the hump in your back and your distended stomach don't allow you to wear your normal size. You feel that all you are left to wear are "dumpy" clothes that hang like tents. After you make your purchase, your friend assists you to the local restaurant. You arrive out of breath and feeling like you have just "had it" for the day. Your poor posture not only compresses your lungs and prevents normal breathing, but you are left staring at the floor as you walk. No matter how much your friend keeps jabbering away, you feel cut off from the rest of the world around you. Finally, you arrive home two hours later, exhausted.

## Osteoporosis Risk Factors

You may already have osteoporosis if you have picked up this book. So how can this list of risk factors help you now? There are some risk factors that you cannot change, like genetics. But you may find risk factors on this list that you *can* change. If you are taking part in any habit or activity that is known for reducing bone density, you can make the choice to change that behavior and prevent further bone loss.

▶ **Gender.**

Your chances of developing osteoporosis are greater if you are a woman. Women have less bone tissue and lose bone more rapidly than men because of hormonal changes that take place during menopause.

▶ **Age.**

The older you are, the greater your risk of osteoporosis. Your bones become weaker and less dense as you age. Women experience most of their bone loss during menopause. Men, barring any medical condition, don't lose bone mass until their late 60s to early 70s.

▶ **Body Size.**

Small-boned women are at greater risk of osteoporosis just because there isn't a lot of bone mass to begin with. My sister, who has teeny little wrists that I can loop my thumb and forefinger around twice, is at a higher risk for osteoporosis than I am. I am a much "sturdier" gal, and therefore, at lower risk.

▶ **Ethnicity.**

Caucasian and Asian women are at highest risk. African-American and Hispanic women come in a very close second. A Caucasian woman with fair skin and red or blond hair is considered at highest risk because of the lack of collagen present in her body to begin with. For me—a freckle-faced, former redhead—the odds are not stacked in my favor. For all ethnic groups, calcium intake is much lower than it should be and, therefore, puts all people at considerable risk for the disease. For more information about particular ethnic risks, see Chapter 2.

▶ **Family History.**

Whether or not you'll ever suffer a fracture may be determined by your genes. People whose parents have a history of osteoporosis generally have some of the same predispositions that lead to osteoporosis. But just because a parent may have had broken bones doesn't mean you will. You can prevent it.

▶ **Menopause.**

Dropping estrogen levels, which occur during perimenopause and menopause, are believed to result in bone loss. There is another hormone in the testosterone family—androgen—that slowly begins dropping in women around their mid-20s. It is thought that perhaps the low levels of this hormone that are reached by menopause may be partially responsible for low bone density.

▶ **Amenorrhea.**

Amenorrhea is an absence of menstrual periods in a premenopausal woman. An absence of menses results in low levels of estrogen in a woman's body, which in turn, appears to result in bone loss. Age itself is not the only indicator for bone density in a woman. A young woman experiencing a cessation of menses can have bones like a 70-year-old person with osteoporosis. And just like the osteoporotic 70-year-old, a 20-year-old can have bones that break easily and heal poorly. Amenorrhea, in young women, is generally due to chronic dieting and over-exercising, which both lead to lowered levels of body fat that are too low to support a normal menstrual cycle.

▶ **Hypogonadism.**

Low levels of testosterone in men result in hypogonadism. Just as reduced estrogen appears to result in bone loss in women, the same is true for low levels of testosterone (and possibly estrogen) in men. Approximately 30 percent of men who have suffered a vertebral fracture have sex hormone levels that are below normal. Men do not normally have a sudden drop in sex hormones at middle age the way women do. However, certain medications can cause testosterone levels to diminish at an accelerated rate. See the chart on page 26 titled "Illnesses and Their Treatments Can Lead to Low Bone Density."

▶ **Hyperparathyroidism.**

The parathyroid gland is responsible for regulating the amount of calcium in the blood. Somehow, in patients with hyperparathyroidism, the parathyroid gland mistakenly reads the blood as not having enough calcium. As a result, it releases more and more parathyroid hormone to push up the calcium levels in the blood. The calcium that is pushed into the blood is being taken from the bones, resulting in additional calcium being excreted by the kidneys.

▶ **Crohn's Disease, Colitis, and Inflammatory Bowel Disease (IBD).**

All three of these gastrointestinal disorders greatly reduce the amount of calcium that is capable of being absorbed through the digestive tract. Reduced calcium intake over a long period of time is a significant risk factor for low bone density.

▶ **Hypertension.**

Urinary calcium excretion has been found to be significantly higher in hypertensive individuals. Calcium excretion leaves less calcium available to the bones for new bone formation.

▶ **Anorexia.**

Anorexia is often accompanied by amenorrhea, as well as a thin frame and poor eating habits that result in inadequate calcium intake. This leaves an anorexic with at least three risk factors for osteoporosis, without mentioning any secondary diseases that result from the stress of being malnourished.

▶ **Over-Exercising.**

Over-exercising can lead to dangerously low levels of body fat. If a woman also has amenorrhea, her estrogen levels are further reduced, which leads to low bone density. In addition, people who overexercise are generally on a diet that is deficient in many nutrients—especially calcium. These chronic exercisers/dieters eliminate dairy products as a way to reduce fat in their diet.

▶ **Carbonated Beverages.**

The link here is not the carbonation but the proclivity for people who drink a lot of soda to not drink enough milk or consume the foods needed for proper calcium intake. In order to solve my own addiction for two sodas a day, I drink a glass of water before and a glass of orange juice with calcium within an hour or two after my sodas.

▶ **Caffeine.**

High caffeine intake (three or more cups of coffee per day) can promote bone loss. Surprisingly, though, a healthy link has been found between green or black tea (both contain caffeine) and osteoporosis. Studies have found that people who regularly drink green or black tea have less incidence of low bone density at the hip and spine.

▶ **Bilateral Oophorectomy.**

When a woman has had both ovaries removed, the estrogen and progesterone produced at those sites are also removed. Low levels of estrogen put these women at an immediate risk for osteoporosis, regardless of how old they are when they have the surgery.

▶ **Inactive Lifestyle.**

Use it or lose it—moderate amounts of stress to the joints, acquired from exercise, will increase bone density. Conversely, lack of exercise will promote low bone density. It is a tragedy that many young women have turned away from exercise because they want to be thin. They fear that exercise will add weight and bulk to their bodies. Making sure our children get enough exercise is important to protect them against osteoporosis as adults. They must reach a peak or optimum bone mass by the time they are young adults. If a child has low bone density to begin with, she will not be able to afford to lose very much as an adult. The denser the bone, the less likely that a certain amount of inevitable bone loss will lead to osteoporosis.

▶ **Bed rest or Immobility.**

With a long period of immobility, bone density quickly diminishes. It is imperative to get moving as soon as possible after an injury or illness. If it is feasible, bring some hand weights to your bedside.

▶ **Smoking.**

Let's face it, smoking is on every list. Current research reveals that nicotine and other chemicals found in cigarettes may be directly toxic to bone. In addition, smoking may inhibit absorption of calcium and other important nutrients that increase overall health, as well as pre-vent osteoporosis. What researchers do know for sure is that there is a direct link between smoking, rapid bone loss, and a high rate of hip and vertebral fractures.

▶ **Alcohol.**

Heavy drinking of alcoholic beverages can result in hormonal de-ficiencies in both men and women (talk to your doctor about what defines heavy drinking—it may be less than you think). In women, chronic drinking can result in irregular menstrual cycles, an occurrence that increases osteoporosis risk. Alcoholic men tend to produce low testosterone levels. Low testosterone has been linked to a decreased activity of osteoblasts—the cells that stimulate bone formation. On top of all that, alcoholics have been shown to have high levels of cortisol, a corticosteroid. Excessive levels of cortisol have been linked to decreased bone formation and increased bone resorption. Corticosteroids also impair calcium absorption, which leads to an increase in parathyroid hormone secretion (see hyperparathyroidism, page 20).

▶ **Lupus.**

Most lupus patients take a glucocorticoid for the pain, but glucocorticoids are also known for reducing bone density. Studies also show that bone loss may be occurring as a result of the disease itself. Furthermore, bone loss can occur just out of pure inactivity. Many lupus patients are just in too much pain to exercise when the disease is flaring up. Lupus patients need to be vigilant about getting enough vitamin D in order to be able to absorb calcium. Most people get their vitamin D through exposure to sunlight. Many lupus patients usually cannot tolerate the sun and fear a flare-up caused by the sun.

▶ **Fibromyomata.**

Just as with the lupus patients above, many people with fibromyomata are just in too much pain to exercise. Even short periods of inactivity can quickly lead to low bone density. Long periods of inactivity can be disastrous for bone density. If you have fibromyomata, just do as much as you can.

▶ **Hypercalciuria.**

People with this disorder excrete too much calcium through the urine. If the blood loses calcium to the kidneys, there is no way for new bone formation to occur. This means that as old bone is being reabsorbed into the bloodstream, no new bone is being formed—leaving the bones less and less dense all the time. Men are twice as likely to suffer from hypercalciuria than women.

▶ **Osteogenesis Imperfecta.**

Osteogenesis Imperfecta is a genetic disorder characterized by bones that break easily for no apparent cause, thus it is related to osteoporosis.

▶ **Depression.**

The link of depression to osteoporosis is not entirely clear. Scientists initially thought that people with osteoporosis were understandably depressed. After all, chronic disease, coupled with pain, immobility, and potential deformity, would cause depression. However, recent findings suggest that hormone levels influenced by depression might contribute to osteoporosis. There is a higher level of cortisol in the system of a depressed person, which may be causing bone loss. A study also revealed that depressed women with osteoporosis were more prone to falling and had higher vertebral and non-vertebral (wrist, hip) fractures than their mentally healthy counterparts.

► **Glucocorticoid Use.**

Used predominantly for inflammatory or autoimmune diseases (see the chart on page 26 titled "Illnesses and Their Treatments Can Lead to Low Bone Density"), glucocorticoids (also called steroids) are the most common cause of drug-induced osteoporosis. Steroids lower the quantity of calcium that is able to be absorbed by the intestines. Steroids also increase calcium excretion through the kidneys. The resulting reduction of calcium throughout the body activates the parathyroid glands to increase their secretion of parathyroid hormone (PTH). The PTH is saying, "WHOA! Not enough calcium circulating in the bloodstream. Guess I'll take it from the bones." As if matters weren't bad enough for your calcium levels, the increased PTH results in increased bone breakdown, or resorption. Unfortunately, that's not all the bad news. Glucocorticoid consumption also decreases levels of estrogen and testosterone—important managers of bone metabolism in both men and women. The resultant dwindling estrogen and testosterone are associated with bone loss. On top of that, steroids also cause muscle weakness which will discourage the steroid-user from exercising, resulting in even more bone loss. Last, but far from least, glucocorticoids impact bone directly by stifling bone formation. There is one light in this dark tunnel: If you or a child you know is taking an inhaled steroid, it appears to have no effect on bone density when taken in moderate doses.

## Osteoporosis and Low Bone Density Found at a Disturbing Rate in Young Women

Lori Turner, of the University of Arkansas, recently tested the bone density of 164 young college women. The results were quite unsettling. Two percent of those young women had osteoporosis, another 15 percent had osteopoenia, or low bone density. What does this mean for the future of this disease? Will osteoporosis be more prevalent 20 or 30 years from now? Through my own unscientific observations of the exercise and diet habits of my studio clientele, I would venture to say yes.

In my own studio, my clients in their 60s or older are generally stronger than my younger clients. And when it comes to osteoporosis, *strength matters*. Bone responds to exercise by laying down more material where the extra strength is needed, thus, creating denser bone. I was initially surprised that my older clients were so much stronger, but now I expect it. Although there are more young people with gym memberships than ever before, not all of the memberships result in participation. Many of my younger clients come nowhere near accomplishing the amount of exercise my grandmother and even my mother obtained in their everyday lives as children and young adults. They didn't go to a gym, but life in general was more active. The other interesting fact is that my grandmother didn't show signs of low bone density until she was in her late 70s, while my mother has osteopoenia and is only in her early 60s. Could that be due to the fact that my grandmother's young life lacked the luxuries that my mother had? And if so, I had a lot more luxuries and got less exercise because of it than my mother. Where does that leave me and my generation? Does that leave us with a higher risk of osteoporosis?

Lori Turner's study turned up some interesting habits of her test subjects that are very prevalent among young women. Some of her subjects had extremely low body weights, maintained exclusively through dieting. These young women were avoiding exercise completely because they didn't want to "bulk up." These young women also eliminated dairy products because of their fat content—excluding much needed calcium for reaching peak bone mass, which usually occurs in young adulthood. At the opposite end of the spectrum, Turner found that young women who had participated in high school sports had the highest bone density scores. This goes along with well-accepted data that shows that moderate amounts of exercise increases bone density.

If I had the opportunity to speak to the young women who aren't exercising and whose eating habits are abominable, I would probably begin by impressing on them the importance of quality of life. If you do absolutely nothing in the way of exercise, then you can expect the aches and pains of old age to begin at a very young age. Discomfort usually begins in the shoulders but sometimes the low back. I would ask them, "If you don't even go for a few walks every week, how can you possibly have the energy to spend a day at a museum, at a concert, at an amusement park, or site-seeing on vacation?" I think dragging a 20-year-old around for the day who just doesn't have the energy to sustain a normal day's activities would be pretty darn sad, but not unheard of when I think of the 20-somethings that I have taught. I taught a few dance classes a couple of years ago at a local community college and was appalled at the lack of strength these young women exhibited. Even "girlie" push-ups were out of the question.

As far as poor diet, I would tell them that having been a dancer, I probably had worse eating habits than they can even imagine having and that I am paying for it now. My once perfect teeth have cavities. My normally simple and cramp-free menstrual cycle was accompanied by a two-week migraine every month for about two years. I also have hypoglycemia, which makes me susceptible to diabetes. If they appear to show signs of anorexia or bulimia, I would tell them that they are wrecking havoc with their metabolism. Their bodies are starving, and the more they starve their bodies, the greater their bodies are going to hang on to every small calorie they ingest. If and when they are ever ready to stop the binge-and-starve cycle, they could easily gain 20 pounds on a 1,200 calorie diet. I did a great

## Illnesses and Their Treatments
## Can Lead to Low Bone Density

| Illness | Medications | Common Examples |
|---|---|---|
| Asthma, Chronic Obstructive Pulmonary Disease, Osteoarthritis, Crohn's Disease, Inflammatory Bowel Syndrome, Ulcerative Colitis, Psoriasis, Lupus, Cystic Fibrosis, Rheumatoid Arthritis, Psoriasis, Pulmonary Fibrosis | Glucocorticoids, Cortisone, Hydrocortisone, Prednisone, Dexamethasone, Methylprednisolone, Intranasal Corticosteroids, Corticosteroids (This class of drugs causes increased calcium and potassium secretion and can lead to amenorrhea.) | Beconase, Vancenase, Vanceril, Lotrisone, Diprolene, Elecon, DeHasone, Orasone, Azmacort, Nasacort |
| Epilepsy | Anticonvulsants (interfere with Vitamin D absorption) | Cerebyx, Neurontin, Zarontin |
| Gastrointestinal Disorders | Antacids containing aluminum. | Alu-tab, Basaljel, Alujel, Amphojel |
| Cancer, Immune System Disorders, Neoplastic Disease, Rheumatoid Arthritis, Psoriasis | Chemotherapy, Methotrexate | Rheumatrex, Trexall |
| High Cholesterol | Cholestyramine (impairs absorption of many nutrients) | Questran, Questran Light |
| Water Retention | Loop diuretics (causes loss of potassium and magnesium, which help the body to absorb calcium) | Bumex, Adecrin, Lasix, Demadex |
| Endometriosis | GRH analogs (some women are treated simultaneously with GRH analog and an osteoporosis treatment) | Lupron, Supprelin, Synarel, Nafarelin, Zoladex |
| Certain blood vessel, lung, and heart conditions | Heparin (interferes with metabolism of vitamin D—which aids in the absorption of calcium—resulting in an increased risk of bone loss) | Calciparine, Liquaemin |

disservice to my health, despite being physically active, and would hope to make young women understand how incredibly not worthwhile my bad eating habits were. It took many years to recover from my poor eating habits, but now that I am eating like a "normal" person, my quality of life has put me at the top of my game—everyday. Pass this info on to any young people you know. Maybe it will scare them straight.

One last thing from Lori Turner's study—she found a connection between low bone density and the birth control drug, Depo-Provera. The National Institute of Health has also supported a study that resulted in findings of low bone density in women taking Depo-Provera. The drug (a progesterone injection given once every three months) stops a woman's menstrual flow and is very popular with young women. The study revealed that young women taking Depo-Provera had bone densities similar to what you would expect in a postmenopausal woman. The study did show that after stopping Depo-Provera use, bone density did return in time. But what if a young woman was to take this drug for many years? What would happen if she stopped taking the drug after her peak bone building years had passed? Would she be able to build up the surplus density she would need before passing through menopause? These are all questions to which I certainly would want answers before using Depo-Provera.

# Anatomy of a Bone: Living Tissue, Not Inert Concrete

Bone is alive. Bone is not a concrete-like, nonliving structure. Bone not only protects and supports the soft tissues of the body, but it is constantly creating new red blood cells, white blood cells, and platelets. Your bones are alive, moving, and constantly changing. To think that bone is not a living substance is like saying, "Well, those are just the tree's roots. All they do is keep the tree from blowing away." Bones do much more than just keep us from melting into a puddle, which is why they need to be given the same care and attention that we give the rest of our body.

Although we think of bones as being a hard, sturdy, solid material, they actually more closely resemble a complicated system of tunnels with walls made up of collagen and calcium phosphate. In fact, this tunnel system looks very similar to a sponge or a microscopic view of a woven fabric. There is a lot of open space in a healthy bone. In an osteoporotic bone, there is too much space and the woven, intricate system of bone becomes frail.

## Wicker Chairs and Thinning Bone

A healthy bone's framework can be likened to the strong woven pattern in a new wicker chair. The fibers are sturdy, flexible, and resilient, just like healthy bone. Now imagine that chair after years of use. The fibers have become brittle and break easily. Entire fibers on the chair have loosened from the framework, creating holes and weaknesses. This is very similar to what happens to a bone damaged by osteoporosis. There are gaps in the bone tissue where entire parts of the bone have disintegrated. The bone framework that remains looks frayed and much thinner.

It's easy to picture what low bone density looks like if you can picture an old wicker chair compared to a new one.

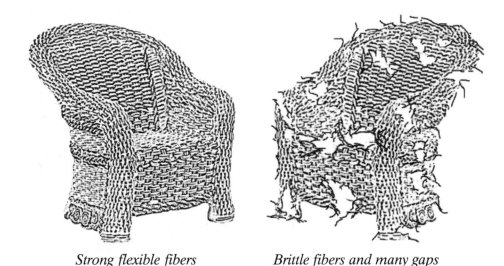

*Strong flexible fibers*               *Brittle fibers and many gaps*

## A Little Experiment

Imagine that our wicker chair from above represents a microscopic view of your bones. (Although, the old bones are actually much more brittle and hard than the old wicker chairs.) Now imagine these two chairs as two pieces of bone from your spine. Imagine simulating a real fall by dropping each piece of bone to the floor. The example on the left is going to fare much better. You may have a small crack or nick in the bone, but that would be all. On the other hand, the example on the right looks as if it would not only break, but shatter, with a lot less force than a fall. In fact, many osteoporosis-related fractures do not need the pressure of a fall in order to break. The pressure can come from doing a sit-up, getting out of bed without first rolling to one side, or even just tying your shoes. There is a full explanation of preventing fracture by avoiding certain postures and movements in Chapter 3.

# What is Osteoporosis?

Osteoporosis finds its roots in Greek, meaning "passages through bones." There are two types of bone: *cortical* (hard) and *cancellous* (spongy). The part of the bone that is most affected by osteoporosis is the spongy bone. The vertebrae of the spine, the hip, and the wrist are most affected by osteoporosis simply because they have a higher percentage of this spongy type of bone. With osteoporosis, the spongy bone at these sites becomes more and more like our worn-out wicker chair, and it is easy to understand how a little bit too much pressure can cause those brittle, thinning fibers to break.

## How Does the Bone Actually Get So Thin?

The thinning of bones occurs when old bone is removed into the bloodstream (resorption) faster than new bone is added (formation). After age 30, bone resorption slowly begins to exceed bone formation. Bone loss becomes rapid in the first few years after menopause but persists into the postmenopausal years. As men and women age, it is assumed that a certain amount of bone density will be lost. Whether or not we develop osteoporosis depends on how much bone mass we lose and how much bone mass we had to begin with. In addition to normal bone loss as a result of aging, osteoporosis can develop whenever bone is resorbed into the bloodstream too quickly or when bone formation occurs too slowly to allow for adequate healthy bone density. The risk factors previously listed can all lead to an imbalance in bone resorption and bone formation that, in turn, can lead to osteoporosis.

### Symptoms of Osteoporosis

| Symptoms | |
|---|---|
| **Usually:** | None |
| **Occasionally:** | Loss of Height<br>Back Pain: which is later diagnosed as a vertebral fracture |

# Getting Tested

Osteoporosis is considered a "silent disease." There are generally no warning signs or symptoms until the disease has advanced or you have experienced a fracture. Please don't forget, as you consider whether or not you should be tested, that fractures can lead to irreversible deformities and that getting tested is *simple*. You must be tested in order to know if you have osteoporosis. There are many different types of bone density tests available to you.

I had my first bone density test when I was 33. It was a quantitative ultrasound performed at the local drugstore. I wanted to get a baseline to see how much my bone density would drop as I got older. I was surprised to find that my bone density was already slightly below average for my age. Having been a professional dancer, and now a personal trainer, I was a bit surprised. Some bad eating habits and over-exercising definitely had caught up with me. But why should *you* get tested? Have your bone density measured if:

1.  You have one or more of the risk factors listed previously in this chapter.

2.  You are postmenopausal.

3.  You have long-term, nagging back pain that you don't feel is due to exercise.

4.  You have a family history of osteoporosis.

5.  You have any broken bones after 40. (I have worked with several premenopausal women with low bone density. One particular client went to the doctor with pain in her ribs. It turned out that she cracked her ribs while using the weight machines at the local gym. She was tested and diagnosed with osteopoenia, or low bone density.)

## It's All About You

In a survey of approximately 559 postmenopausal women, performed by the International Osteoporosis Foundation, the women all said that osteoporosis was a major concern for them as they approached a more mature age. Interestingly enough, only a very small percentage of these women talked to their doctors about preventative measures. Why is that? The only answer that comes to mind is that they just don't think it could happen to them. However, one in two women is a pretty high statistic, and that is for osteoporosis fractures—not for the disease itself. Get checked if you have any doubt. I personally think it should be a routine test for all women who are menopausal. After all, the test is painless and could offer you invaluable information about your health. Remember: Osteoporosis is a debilitating disease, and fractures don't just happen to other people. It's worth your time to take the test.

**Common Tests Available for Bone Mineral Density Testing**

| Tests | Measurement Site |
|---|---|
| Dual Energy X-ray Absorptiometry (DXA). | Spine, hip, or total body. |
| Peripheral Dual Energy X-ray Absorptiometry (pDXA). | Wrist, heel, or finger. |
| Single Energy X-ray Absorptiometry (SXA). | Wrist or heel. |
| Quantitative Ultrasound (QUS). | Heel, shinbone, or kneecap. |
| Dual Photon Absorptiometry (DPA). | Spine or hip. |

# T-Scores, Z-Scores, and SDs: Reading the Results of Your Test

You could end up with two scores on your test—a T-score and a Z-score.

| T-Scores and Z-Scores |
|---|
| **T-Score:** A score that relates your test to what is normal for a young, healthy adult at their peak bone mass. |
| **Z-Score:** A score that relates your results to other people in your age group. |

The "SD" that you see after your number score (-1SD for example) stands for standard deviation. *Standard deviation* is the difference between your bone mineral density and that of a healthy young adult. If you have a score within one standard deviation of the norm, then you are considered to have normal bone density. But if your score reads -1.1 or lower, then you have low bone mass or osteopoenia. Maybe the following chart will make it a little easier to understand.

## SD Scores

| Your Score | What It Means |
|---|---|
| -1SD or higher. | Normal. Low fracture risk. |
| -1.1SD to -2.5 SD. | Low bone density or Osteopoenia. Moderate fracture risk—must follow the *5 Golden Rules* in Chapter 3. |
| Greater than -2.5 SD. | Severe and established osteoporosis. High fracture risk—must follow the *5 Golden Rules* in Chapter 3. |

# Bone Mineral Density Chart

This is a typical graph that you will receive after a bone mineral density test. The graph shows your bone mineral density compared to your age, in order to find your T-score. For the example on page 33, I have used my own bone mineral density test from 2001. The "X" represents where my age and my score intersect. You can see that I am slightly below the national average. Because I am slightly below the National Average line to begin with, I continue to follow the National Average line across the graph while staying slightly below. I find that, as I age, my risk for dropping under the T-line and into the danger zone is low. Many factors (as previously listed) can change that, but for now, I am a low risk for osteoporosis.

## Reading Your Score

Bone Mineral Density Score:  0.521    T-Score:  -0.5

In order to find my score on the chart, I first found my age (33) and made a vertical line up the chart. Next, I found my Bone Mineral Density Score on the left of the graph and made a horizontal line, marking an "X" where the two lines intersect.

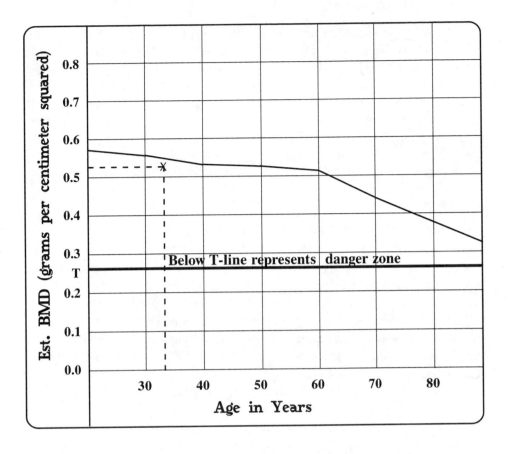

## Men and Osteoporosis

Many people believe that osteoporosis is a disease for women: it simply is not. In 1994, osteoporosis fractures in men accounted for one-fifth of the total expenditure for osteoporosis fractures—almost $3 billion in the United States alone. Approximately one-fourth of all hip fractures occur in men, and of men over the age of 50, one out of every 100 will suffer a hip fracture. So why are men not generally questioned about their potential risk for osteoporosis if they account for almost one-sixth of the $17 billion spent annually on osteoporosis? Shouldn't they be encouraged to have routine bone density tests after a certain age? Or at least be informed about the potential secondary causes of osteoporosis outside of age? The answer is yes, they should. Of course they should. But a questionnaire issued to hundreds of doctors by the International Osteoporosis Foundation showed that, generally, the doctors who participated were not even encouraging *women* to have routine bone density testing or informing them of secondary osteoporosis risk. So why would *men* be informed, if they suffer osteoporosis fractures only *half* as frequently as women? It is true that men are not given a lot of attention in the area of osteoporosis, and that this needs to be changed. Men need to be included in screening and testing for and information about low bone density.

While a heavier skeleton and a lack of rapidly diminishing hormonal levels at mid-life protect many men from early bone loss, their ability to absorb calcium begins to decline somewhere around the age of 66–70. With the number of men over 70 years old expected to double by the year 2050, the concern for osteoporosis in men is growing. In 1999, the National Institute of Health began a seven-year research program to study osteoporosis in men. Scientists hope to discover the largest risk sources of low bone density in men. Presently, though, there are many known factors that cause secondary osteoporosis in men, or osteoporosis that is not due to a mature age (70 and older).

## Secondary Osteoporosis in Men

Secondary osteoporosis is any low bone density not brought on by the usual aging process. I say the *usual* aging process instead of normal aging process because, with a continued and steady exercise program, it might be possible to halt the usual bone loss that occurs with age. Perhaps what contributes to bone loss in men is the fact that we usually are not as active and usually don't exercise as much as we get older. In any case, to find if you are at risk for secondary osteoporosis, go through the list of contributing factors (pages 19–24), and also check the chart titled "Illnesses and Their Treatments Can Lead to Low Bone Density" (page 26) to see if any medicine that you may be taking is listed.

If you have one or more of the risk factors listed, talk to your doctor about getting tested for osteoporosis. If you find you have low bone density, then read on!

# Four-Part Plan for Osteoporosis

Recent studies support the effectiveness of a multifaceted plan for osteoporosis. The four aspects of your plan will include:

1. Diet.

2. Medication.

3. Exercise.

4. Postural and movement awareness for avoiding fracture.

Studies have shown that combining exercise and calcium increases bone density more than either factor alone. The same is true for medication and exercise. The fourth consideration, postural and movement awareness for avoiding fracture, is an often neglected aspect in treating osteoporosis. (You'll find chapters devoted to each of these four facets in treating osteoporosis later in the book.). Follow a four-part plan that includes safe movement techniques, and you will be doing all you can to live a full, independent, and healthy life without fracture.

## Important Warning for Exercising With Osteoporosis

Do not rush straight into your exercise program. While OsteoPilates is created to be safe for those with low bone density, you will first need to learn the movement rules that make it so.

For example, you will not see any sit-ups in your OsteoPilates program. But would you have guessed that you should not bend over to tie your shoes for the same reason that you shouldn't do a sit-up? What's the correlation? Why are both circumstances putting you at equally high risk for fracturing vertebrae? This book would be of little use to you unless the only movements you plan on doing all day are the exercises at the end of this book. And who is going to do that? You have a life to live! If you are the kind of person who takes things into his or her own hands (and obviously you are or you wouldn't have bought this book) you are going to want to learn to avoid fractures while gardening, walking, doing household chores, and any other activities that you love—not just exercise. Statistics show that most fractures occur in the late afternoon in the home. Chances are that most people are not doing their exercise programs at that time.

My intention here is to impress on you, from the very beginning, *not* to start an exercise program until you are aware of what movements cause fractures (as explained in Chapter 3). Just as I said previously, it is a four-part plan for osteoporosis, not a one- or two-part plan, which will bring you the greatest results. You wouldn't keep you car in tip-top condition in order to keep it safe on the road and then not wear your seatbelt, right? So, don't leave anything out and, of course, talk to your doctor before doing anything.

Okay—let's get started. Happy reading and enjoy your OsteoPilates program!

# Chapter 2

# First Things First: Building Bone Density Before Bone Loss and Menopause

It is true that if your mother had osteoporosis, you are at a higher risk for getting it. But that doesn't mean *you* will get osteoporosis. I work with a client whose mother had over a dozen vertebral fractures, and my client (now 65) does not even have low bone density. She made a decision, at a very young age, to do all she could to prevent osteoporosis. She has been active her whole life and it has paid off for her. Best of all she can out-exercise, out-hike, and out-walk almost all of my other clients.

So, you don't have osteoporosis, and you are thinking, "It would be pretty great if I *never* get osteoporosis." Good idea. No—great idea! In the opinion of numerous health specialists, doctors, and physical therapists, osteoporosis is one of the most preventable diseases. As the loss of bone in women at menopause is predictable, prevention is possible and should be on every woman's mind as she approaches her 40s.

## Building Up a Surplus

Every woman should know that, no matter how dense her bones are before menopause, she *will* experience bone loss during menopause. So why not build up a surplus supply now? After all, you put sunscreen on before going out in the sun, get vaccines before traveling, and wash your hands before eating. Why not build bone density *before* menopause? However, before jumping right into a bone-building exercise program designed exclusively for those *without* low bone density, we'll begin with a discussion of menopause. What are its effects on your bones and what can you do to ease your way through a sometimes difficult time?

## Save Your Fat Calories for the Ice Cream

My husband has a great dieting method. (Stick with me here, this is leading back to osteoporosis.) He knows that a healthy diet includes a certain amount of fat calories. So, he eats *extremely* low-fat foods all day long and puts all of his allocated fat calories into one *humongous* bowl of ice cream at the end of the day.

You can also build up your bone density for when you need it. You can start saving a surplus of bone density now so that when you reach menopause—and the inevitable bone loss—you will have a surplus to draw from, leaving you with adequate bone density to prevent fracture (not as fun as my husband's dieting methods, but if my husband doesn't budget his calories, he'll get fat). If you don't gain bone density early, you will be one of the 50 percent of women in America with a bone fracture due to osteoporosis.

# Menopause

Menopause, a part of every woman's reproductive life cycle, is not generally greeted with enthusiasm. Unlike childbirth or pregnancy, women don't compare "war stories" nearly as freely on the subject of perimenopause or menopause. That leaves younger women not only uninformed, but not even knowing what questions to ask. When I gave birth to my son, no one told me there was an afterbirth…I thought I was done. How was I supposed to know to ask that question? I assumed everything happened at once. Not only was I—a college graduate—a *bit* uninformed, but I was feeling pretty darn stupid.

The situation is similar for most women going through menopause. Most women have heard about the hot flashes and the cessation of menses, but what about the urinary tract infections or vaginal dryness? What about crazy hormonal swings, loss of libido, problems sleeping, and loss of collagen that decreases your skin's smooth appearance? And, of course, what about bone loss and the accompanied loss of height? **Yikes!** No wonder women don't want to talk about menopause…

## You Are Not Alone

It may comfort you to know that you are certainly not alone when passing through menopause. Almost 2 million American women turn 50 each year (the average age for menopause), and 1 in 3 American women are past menopause.

# Where Are You in Relation to Menopause?

Since we are starting with "First Things First," let's look at where you are in your reproductive life before considering menopausal symptoms.

To get an idea of where you are in relation to menopause, you can ask your doctor to order a test. In addition, there are also easy over-the-counter urine tests that have recently become available to the American market. Just like the doctor-ordered test, the home test reads your level of follicle-stimulating hormone (FSH). The pituitary gland in the brain produces FSH, which in turn encourages the ovaries to develop and release eggs. An increase in FSH may mean a decline in fertility. Therefore, if FSH is elevated, you may be moving towards menopause. It is essential to speak with your physician about the results of these home tests.

## Increased Hormones and Declining Fertility

Doesn't quite make sense, does it? It seems that a high level of hormones should mean more reproduction capability. Actually, your pituitary gland is producing more FSH in order to keep your body's estrogen at its usual level. The more FSH, the less estrogen your ovaries are producing.

## Reproductive Life Cycle of Women

Researchers have defined stages, in order to more accurately determine exactly where a woman is in relation to menopause. The designations exclude smokers, obese, or overly thin women, as well as women who have irregular menses. Very athletic women who do a lot of aerobic exercise are also excluded from these designations.

| | |
|---|---|
| **Peak Reproductive:** | Regular menses, FSH is normal. |
| **Early Perimenopause:** | Regular menses, FSH levels begin to rise. |
| **Mid Perimenopause:** | Somewhat irregular menses (off schedule by up to a week and a half), FSH increases. |
| **Late Perimenopause:** | Irregular menses (up to two months without a menstrual period), FSH is elevated. |
| **Menopause:** | Menopause is a 12-month cessation of menstrual periods. |
| **Early Menopause:** | The first four years after menopause occurs, FSH is elevated. |
| **Late Postmenopause:** | Lasts until death, FSH is elevated. |

# What's Happening to My Body?

Now that you have an idea as to where you are in relation to menopause, let's look at your body's response to the changes that may be happening.

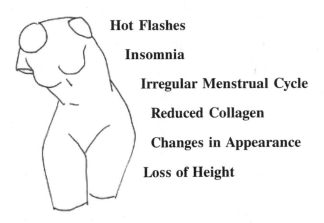

Hot Flashes

Insomnia

Irregular Menstrual Cycle

Reduced Collagen

Changes in Appearance

Loss of Height

## Irregular Menstrual Cycles

Changes in menses are often the first sign of mid perimenopause. Your period could become lighter, heavier, longer, or shorter. Changing levels of the sex hormone progesterone have a lot to do with the changes you may be experiencing. The job of progesterone is to get your uterus ready for the arrival of a fertilized egg. If an egg is not fertilized, progesterone is the hormone in charge of shedding the thickened lining of the uterus. When the ovaries do not manufacture enough progesterone to shed the lining, the lining will continue to grow until your estrogen levels drop enough to bring on a menses. Heavy bleeding often results if a menstrual cycle occurs after the lining has had two or three months to thicken.

## Hot Flashes

The most common sign of early, mid, or late perimenopause, approximately 75 percent of Caucasian women experience hot flashes. A hot flash can cause a slight feeling of warmth or enough heat to soak your clothes. They can also be bad enough to interfere with your sleep, which leads to insomnia (next on our list of menopausal symptoms). Some women are able to pinpoint a trigger that brings on their hot flashes. You may be able to avoid that situation. Some triggers include: hot drinks, stress, spicy foods, caffeine, and alcohol. Remedies for hot flashes may include dressing in layers (especially when you are going to exercise), keeping your bedroom cool, and drinking ice water. Supplements recommended for hot flashes, or hormone replacement, have also been known to help women who are suffering from hot flashes. Hormone replacement therapy (HRT) came under close scrutiny in 2002 with the finding of a study called The Women's Health Initiative. This study, along with hormone replacement therapy, is discussed in length in Chapter 5. Early studies of fluoxetine and paroxetine, both antidepressants, have shown that they may be possible future treatments for hot flashes.

## Insomnia

Interrupted sleeping patterns don't make dealing with perimenopausal symptoms any easier. For some women, insomnia is caused by hot flashes that occur at night and result in night sweats. Other women are awakened by the need to go to the bathroom. Either way, going back to sleep can be a problem or, for some, getting to sleep in the first place is the main problem.

## Vaginal and Urinary Tract Changes

The decreased amount of fatty tissue and collagen and decreased blood flow, as we approach menopause, affects the vaginal tissues. The skin of the vagina becomes thinner and drier and the vagina is secreting less mucus. These decreases are due to aging and the changing levels of estrogen. Consequently, the vaginal tissues become more delicate and susceptible to tearing and infection. Intercourse may be uncomfortable, or even painful, as a result. Those women suffering during intercourse could try a water-based lubricant—*not* petroleum jelly. Besides vaginal infections, urinary tract infections are not uncommon during perimenopause. Urinary leakage can also be a problem for some women as they approach menopause.

## Libido

Lack of interest in sex, accompanied by the inability to be aroused, affects some women during perimenopause. For a number of women, it is simply too uncomfortable. There also seems to be a concern among the researchers of libido and menopause that there may be underlying psychological issues that a woman may be dealing with that are affecting her interest in sex. It may not be the hormonal changes but the thought of getting older that is interfering with her desire to be intimate. Although menopause is not considered to mark the nearing end of a woman's life (as it used to, a century or so ago), it often marks the end of a certain way of life. As many women approach menopause, they are also sending children off to college and beginning to grapple with reentering the work force or becoming more involved in work, now that they have more time.

As an interesting note that you don't hear very often, not all women struggle with libido during menopause. For some, their libido actually increases because they no longer have to worry about becoming pregnant.

## Physical Changes

Either as a result of perimenopause or just from getting older, you will notice changes in your body. You might experience a thickening around your waist. You could lose muscle mass and gain more fatty tissue. Your skin might become thinner and lose its elasticity. These changes don't sound terribly appealing but at least the increased fat has hormonal benefits as well. A little extra fat helps a woman's body to continue producing estrogen, which will in turn help to reduce the affects of some menopausal symptoms.

## Memory

Memory problems may simply be an issue of growing older. Middle-aged women and men commonly report short-term memory problems. Whether changing estrogen levels cause the memory problems is unknown, but research has shown that the brain is sensitive to the effects of estrogen. The good news is that memory seems to respond well to exercise, just like our muscles respond to exercise. Challenge your memory with a new game, such as chess; a new skill, such as weaving; or by taking a class that you've never had time for in the past. Research has proven that your effort will be repaid by an improved memory. If you don't use it, you lose it.

## Emotions

Mood swings, depression, and irritability are common during perimenopause. When looking at a chart that portrays rising and falling hormone levels, a premenopausal woman's hormone levels are regular and predictable. The perimenopausal woman looks like she is going through hell. The rise and fall of normal hormones is about as predictable as the up and down motion of a steadily dribbled basketball, while a chart that portrays perimenopausal hormones more closely resembles a rubber ball bouncing madly around a five-foot cell. There are long peaks of high hormone levels that lower slightly, only to shoot wildly back up the chart. With a regular menstrual cycle, it is easy to predict when premenstrual irritability, bloating, or pain may occur. During perimenopause, you may not experience one or two days of a premenstrual-like syndrome but perhaps a full week. It is also impossible to predict the rise and fall of hormonal levels in a perimenopausal woman. Hence, one period may not come for two or three months, followed by a period that lasts two weeks. Grrrrr...I can't remember—what is it that *men* have to deal with at middle age?

## Bone Loss and Prevention

The bone loss that you will experience in the years just following menopause will be the most drastic drop in bone mineral density that you will experience. The rapid drop is a result of decreased estrogen levels. Unlike the other menopausal symptoms, you won't feel a thing as your bones decrease in density. You won't be in pain, and you will feel no discomfort or irritability due to the bone loss. Bone loss is too often pushed to the back burner of concern as women are faced with more pressing and, sometimes, even painful symptoms of menopause. Don't allow this to happen to you. It is easy to take a calcium supplement, and the exercises that you'll be doing to prevent bone loss will aid your other menopausal symptoms.

Some women who are at high risk may also consider taking a preventative medication. Studies have revealed that doctors and premenopausal women agree that osteoporosis is definitely one of the top concerns of aging, but *prevention* is often neglected. In a survey conducted by the International Osteoporosis Foundation, only 6 percent of the women interviewed, who do not have osteoporosis, are taking a preventative medication. Approximately 78 percent said they would take preventative measures if their doctors recommended it. So while osteoporosis fractures are a major health concern for women and their doctors, it looks like some information may be falling into a communication gap. Many women don't know about preventative therapy and they need to seek more open communication with their doctors concerning prevention therapy options. The survey also revealed that most doctors do not prescribe medication for osteoporosis until there has already been a fracture. Since bone density increases much more readily before having osteoporosis, let alone a fracture, preventative measures need to be considered more carefully.

## Your Hormones, Menopause, and Bone Loss

We discussed the role of follicle-stimulating hormone earlier in this chapter, but there are three other hormones that play a big role in the changes associated with menopause. The levels of the hormones estrogen, progesterone, and androgen will be fluctuating during perimenopause and producing changes in your body as you approach menopause. These hormones are secreted by several of the many glands in your body that are part of the endocrine system. Androgen, estrogen, and progesterone help to regulate metabolism, growth, and reproduction. They also play an important role in bone health.

The hormones that regulate the changes leading to menopause are produced by several glands and organs that, as a whole, make up the endocrine system. These hormonal changes generate a considerable effect on bone density.

### Estrogen and Bone Loss

The term *estrogen* actually refers to three hormones: estradiol, estrone, and estriol. It is believed that a falling level of estradiol is most responsible for the rapid bone loss that occurs in the 5–7 years following menopause. Ovary production of estradiol can slow down 5–10 years before

## The Endocrine System

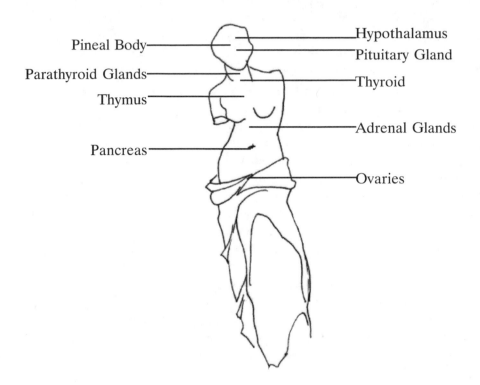

Pineal Body — Hypothalamus
Parathyroid Glands — Pituitary Gland
Thymus — Thyroid
Pancreas — Adrenal Glands
— Ovaries

true menopause. This would affect the body's ability to maintain or build bone density. While it is never too late to increase bone density, a woman's ability to build bone density decreases after menopause. Bone mineral density can certainly be increased after menopause, but your bones will respond much more rapidly before menopause.

A weaker hormone—estrone—continues to be produced in fat tissues and increases with age and fatty tissue. If you gain weight during menopause, it may be your body's way of trying to help you produce more estrone. In a study at the University of California at San Francisco, researchers found that some women whose bodies produce even modest amounts of estrogen after menopause have more protection from hip or spine fracture after the age of 65 than women who have undetectable levels of estrogen in their blood.

It is clear that our own estrogen has many protective benefits, but what about estrogen replacement therapy in the form of prescription drugs? There are many wide-ranging positive effects of estrogen replacement therapy for menopausal symptoms, including not only maintenance of bone density, but also relief from vaginal dryness, fewer mood swings, and diminishing hot flashes and night sweats. Because 50 percent of American women over the age of 50 will experience an osteoporosis fracture, estrogen depletion at menopause is a factor that needs serious attention.

## Androgen and Bone Loss

Androgens are generally thought of as male hormones. However, females do produce them. These androgens are now coming under closer inspection as an option in hormone replacement therapy, especially as combined with estrogen replacement therapy.

A woman's ovaries and adrenal glands produce notable amounts of androgens in the form of testosterone, androstenedione, DHEA (dehydroepiandrosterone), and DHT (dihydrotestosterone). Androgens are thought to contribute to a woman's sexual function, bone health, muscle tone, mood, and energy level. Unlike estrogen, which declines rapidly at menopause, androgens begin declining around the age of 30. By the time menopause rolls around, androgen levels will have already dropped 50 percent from what they were in a woman's 20s. Research is presently being conducted to find out if androgen replacement therapy will be a feasible method of treatment for alleviating certain menopausal symptoms. Some of these early studies have shown that androgen is effective for strengthening bones and muscles and for reducing body fat. Over-the-counter androgens such as DHEA supplements are available, but side-effects can include acne, facial hair, lowered voice, liver injury, fluid retention, sleep apnea, aggressive behavior, and a lowering of HDH cholesterol (the good cholesterol). As with all supplements, DHEA is not regulated by the Food and Drug Administration, so beware—some of these supplements may contain too little DHEA to be effective or too much to be safe.

# Alternative Treatments: Botanicals and Complementary Medicine

Alternative medical treatments are receiving more and more interest due to their more "natural" way of treating menopause. Many women feel that since menopause is not a disease, it should not be treated like one. Other women fear side effects of hormone replacement therapy drugs. Some women are looking for safe and gentle ways to treat their menopausal symptoms and promote bone health, which do not include taking a prescription drug. Alternative treatments can be broken down into two main categories: botanicals and complementary medicine.

## Botanicals

Botanicals include food and supplements derived from any plant part. They are not called herbs because "herbal" refers only to supplements made from the leaves and stems of a plant.

### Supplement Warning

The supplements listed in the table on pages 46 and 47 are listed for informational purposes only. You *must* speak with a physician before add-

## Botanical Treatments for Menopausal Symptoms

| Botanical | Traditional Uses | Known Side Effects |
| --- | --- | --- |
| Angelica or Dong Quai | Menopausal symptoms. | Anticoagulant (should not be taken with other anticoagulants, such as Heparin), photosensitivity. |
| Anise | Menopausal symptoms. | |
| Black Cohosh | Hot flashes, night sweats. | Nausea, vomiting. |
| Calcium | Osteoporosis protection. | |
| Chamomile | Insomnia. | |
| Chasteberry (or Vitex) | Vaginal dryness, depression, libido. | Antiandrogenic effects. |
| DHEA (an androgen called an anti-aging miracle drug) | Menopausal symptoms. | In women: acne, facial hair, menstral changes, aggressive behavior, liver injury, fluid retention, could speed up T-cell decline. |
| Evening Primrose | Hot flashes, irritability. | |
| Ginseng | Fatigue, libido. | Hypertension, insomnia, depression. |
| Ipriflavone | Osteoporosis protection, hormone balance, hot flashes. | Suppression of lymphocytes or immune system. |
| Licorice | Estrogenic activity for hormone balance, hot flashes. | Avoid if you have high blood pressure. |
| Magnesium | Osteoporosis protection. | Too much magnesium from supplements may cause diarrhea. |
| Phosphorous | Osteoporosis protection. | Most people do not need a phosphorous supplement, as this mineral is an additive in many foods. |

## Botanical Treatments for Menopausal Symptoms

| Botanical | Traditional Uses | Known Side Effects |
|---|---|---|
| Potassium | Bone health. | |
| Red Clover | Hot flashes, night sweats. | |
| SAM-e | Mild depression. | |
| Saw Palmetto | Urinary tract infection. | Antiandrogenic (androgens are hormones that play a key role in sexuality and prevent bone loss and increase bone density). |
| Soy and Flaxseed products (Phytoestrogens, which are plant sterols that exert estrogenic activity) | Hot flashes, night sweats, vaginal dryness, dyspareunia (pain during intercourse). | Anticoagulant (should not be taken with other anticoagulants, such as Heparin). |
| St. John's Wort | Mild depression. | Side effects similar to, but much less pronounced than, prescription antidepressants, such as Zoloft and Celexa. |
| UvaUrsi (bearberry) | Urinary tract and bladder health. | Tinnitus, vomiting, seizures. |
| Valerian | Insomnia. | Dystonic reactions resembling partial seizures, visual impairments. |
| Vitamin D | Osteoporosis protection (aids calcium absorption). | Dystonic reactions. |
| Vitamin K | Prevents calcium depletion from bones. | Stored in fatty tissues and potentially toxic in high doses. |
| Wild Mexican Yam (a natural source of DHEA) | (See "DHEA" entry). | |

ing a supplement to your diet. Supplements, either by themselves or in combination with a preexisting condition or traditional medical pharmaceutical, may cause severe adverse side effects.

# Complementary Medicine

Anything outside the mainstream medical practice is currently referred to as *complementary medicine*. Complementary medicine is a field that is continuing to receive more attention and consideration. In fact, the National Institute of Health has created a new division for the sole purpose of studying alternatives to traditional medicine. As increasing amounts of money are spent each year on alternative care rather than on traditional healthcare, the need for proven results has grown. Unfortunately, the jury is still out on most alternative methods of treatment. Although there exists a host of complementary methodologies, we'll be looking at two in particular, for treating menopausal symptoms: acupuncture and reiki. I chose these two forms because of my direct experience with them and the positive results that they yielded. For me, they were both very effective for alleviating pain.

## Acupuncture

Acupuncture is one of the few forms of complementary medicine that has gained acceptance from the Food and Drug Administration and from a panel of scientific experts from the National Institute of Health. A study by Dr. Abass Alavi, of the University of Pennsylvania Hospital, found measurable changes in the brain regions that perceive pain. In fact, because of this proof, many insurance companies now cover acupuncture visits— an important consideration when looking for alternative healthcare.

With a history that can be traced back approximately 2,500 years, acupuncture has long been an important part of Chinese medicine and, in recent years, has gained popularity in the United States. Acupuncture methods are based on the theory that the body has natural paths of energy flow. This energy is referred to as Qi or Chi. Undeterred energy, flowing throughout the body, results in good health. If the energy patterns become disordered or blocked, then disease occurs. Acupuncture restores healthy energy flow to restore health in the individual.

Acupuncture methods include using disposable needles that are sometimes hooked up to electronic stimulation. The needles are inserted into the skin or muscle at specific pressure points. There is also *acupressure*, which is a manual, hands-on treatment without the use of needles. (For example, the pressure point for headaches is the dip between the thumb and the first finger. An acupressure practitioner would press on this point to relieve a headache.) Treatments last approximately 30 minutes.

I had migraines that were lasting up to two and a half weeks every month for which I received acupuncture treatment. My practitioner, Sepideh Lackpour of Santa Clarita, California, used needles, not acupressure.

I found it fascinating that there were points on my body at which I could not feel the needles at all. There were other places on my body that felt very tingly and somewhat painful. These points changed from visit to visit. Eventually, though, the tingling subsided entirely as the energy was balanced. While I usually walked out of the office feeling rather light-headed (which is normal), I always felt better than when I went in. My migraines would generally subside but not always go away completely.

Sepideh had this to add about acupuncture for menopausal symptoms:

"Gynecological problems have been treated with acupuncture for over 200 years, and for 5000 years with herbal medicine. Chinese medicine takes into account the whole pattern of each patient's physical, mental, and emotional symptoms. This is the secret to treating menopause. There are many different herbal formulas that address various symptoms of menopause—from physical ones, such as hot flashes, night sweats, insomnia, etc., to mental ones, such as irritability, anxiety, and depression. Acupuncture is used to balance the body fluids, reduce the heat sensations, and calm the mind. Acupuncture and Chinese herbs also address symptoms, such as memory loss, osteoporosis, circulatory problems, sexual difficulties, and digestive problems, that a woman may encounter during menopause."

## Reiki

*Reiki* means "universal life force energy". Reiki, similar to acupuncture, works on the body's energy paths, or chakra systems, and Chi. During a treatment, the practitioner puts his or her hands on the client in order to restore healthy energy flow.

My experience with reiki for treating migraines was extremely positive. After my first treatment, I felt light-headed but no different. I was disappointed. My practitioner, Sue Ann Nelson of Santa Clarita, California, told me that it may take a few hours to work and sometimes the symptoms get worse before they get better. Sure enough, my migraine went from bad to raging in a matter of hours, but I woke up the next morning without a migraine. Before this first visit, my migraine was already two weeks old, and I thought that perhaps the subsidence was just a coincidence—its time was almost up anyway.

The following month, right before my period started, I got another migraine. I called my practitioner immediately. My headache didn't get worse this time, but it was gone again the next morning. After six or seven months of 2 treatments per month, I no longer got migraines. In fact, with the migraines, I could have never written this book because looking at the computer was just too painful. Any practitioner who manipulates Chi will tell you: When you are balanced, you will be at your very best—able to achieve what you had previously only been able to peripherally consider.

Sue Ann had this to add about reiki:

"Reiki balances the energy systems, and by doing that, harmony is brought to everything [within your body]. Reiki opens the meridian systems that allow everything to have more life force energy. Life force energy is the energy that we are made of, that supports our body. Reiki brings that energy in and releases the energy that is not supporting our system. Reiki also raises the body's vibration level; a healthier body has a higher vibration level."

Sue Ann was always adamant that it was not she who was doing the work but that she was only a facilitator of restoring the health that my body already had and intuitively knew how to restore or bring back to the surface. She insisted that if the universe (or God) can exist in all of the perfection with which it exists, then healing a migraine is a small task. She would also say, "Soon you'll have perfect health," which, at first, made me very skeptical of working with her. I never believed that I would feel really good again. She was right, though—I feel great.

"I don't do the healing, I bring in the energy and it goes where it needs to go. The energy is divinely directed."

—Sue Ann Nelson

# Menopause by Ethnicity: Specific Information Just for You

There's a lot we can learn from each other, even when it comes to the way we culturally and genetically approach menopause.

## Hispanic

Hispanic women tend to go through menopause at an earlier age (the average age is 50) and report urinary leakage more often than other groups. Also, Latinas, regardless of age, consume less calcium than the recommended dietary allowance, making bone loss a greater concern at menopause.

## African-American

In a Study of Women's Health Across the Nation (SWAN), supported by the National Institute of Health, African-American women were found to have the most positive attitude about menopause. They experience more symptoms such as hot flashes, but fewer difficulties with stiffness, headache, and insomnia, when compared to other ethnic groups. In relation to osteoporosis, African-Americans tend to have heavier, denser bones, which initially put them in a lower-risk group for contracting the disease. As they age, their risk for hip fracture doubles approximately every seven years.

Secondary osteoporosis (osteoporosis that is *not* a result of menopause) is a concern for African-Americans because they are susceptible to sickle-cell anemia and lupus (two diseases that are linked to osteoporosis).

## Caucasian

Of Caucasian women, 75 percent suffer from hot flashes. This ethnic group is at highest risk for osteoporosis. Caucasians are also most likely to use postmenopausal hormones. This may be in an effort to reduce their risk of osteoporosis.

## Asian

Asian women report fewer menopausal symptoms—especially hot flashes—than any other ethnic group. While symptoms are low, Asian women also report the most negative feelings toward menopause. Since Asian women, along with Caucasians, are at highest risk for osteoporosis, bone density monitoring is essential. Calcium consumption from alternate sources also needs special attention because many Asian women are lactose intolerant, so they avoid dairy products and don't get the recommended dietary allowance of calcium.

# Eat Your Soy for Reduced Hot Flashes

Studies have linked an Asian diet high in soy products to the reduction of menopausal symptoms. A typical Asian diet contains an average of 40-80 mg of active isoflavones—a phytoestrogen—per day.

## What's a Phytoestrogen?

A phytoestrogen is a plant product that reacts with the body by creating estrogen-like activity. So when estrogen is decreasing at menopause, a phytoestrogen can encourage the endocrine system to produce more estrogen. While in-depth studies still need to be performed, the benefits of phytoestrogens are believed to be most apparent among Asian women, who do not feel the symptoms of menopause as heavily as other populations, believed to be due to the high quantity of plant estrogens that they are consuming daily, mostly in the form of soy. The typical American and European diet contains far less isoflavones than the Asian diet. Many women have recently been implementing soy into their diets for relief of menopausal symptoms, especially hot flashes. If you are interested in increasing your phytoestrogens, check the nutritional values listed on soy products. Most makers of soy products know that people are interested in the amount of active isoflavones in their products and the milligrams can usually be found on the side of the product. The table that follows is the result of a little grocery store researching.

## Soy Products Have Phytoestrogens, Which Have Isoflavones

| Food Item | Milligrams of Active Isoflavones Per Serving |
|---|---|
| Edamame (frozen soybeans, found next to the other frozen vegetables) | 50 mg |
| Tofu | 30 mg |
| Soy milk | 35 mg |
| Raw soybeans (found with the nuts) | 40 mg |
| Soy granola (breakfast cereal) | 20 mg |
| Miso | 35 mg |

# Menopausal Symptoms Are Temporary— Except for Bone Loss

Fortunately, the hot flashes, mood swings, and erratic menstrual cycle will eventually cease. The long-term concern of menopause, however, is bone loss. Bone loss and its accompanying fractures can change the picture of your future considerably. For many people, osteoporosis has meant deformity, debilitation, and life in a nursing home. There is so much information and medication available for preventing bone loss that an osteoporotic fracture shouldn't be a part of any person's future. Demand to have your bone density tested while you are still young so preventative measures can be taken if need be. I say "demand" because I have had several clients request to have their bone density tested, only to be told by their doctors that a bone density scan isn't done until a woman is in her 60s. (Where's the prevention in that?)

When one of my clients in her early 40s was having a lot of upper back pain, I encouraged her to get a bone density test. Her doctor would not order it but ordered an x-ray instead. He called her a couple of days later to tell her that the x-ray showed low bone density and that she would have to have the actual bone density test done.

I have heard it said that you are only as old as your spine. I completely agree. I have a 72-year-old client who can exercise circles around me on the days when my back is being cranky from the years of abuse it endured when I was dancing. On those days, who is the older woman? And how about you? Do you want to age prematurely as the result of spinal fractures? As you age, there's a good chance you'll have enough changes to deal with anyway, without throwing osteoporosis into the mix. Just focus on how you want to live when you "grow up." Get tested, exercise, and take any preventative measures that need to be taken, and you will be kayaking, hiking, gardening, and doing whatever you love for a very long time.

**Chapter 3**

## Not One More Broken Bone: *Preventing Osteoporosis Fractures*

## Fracture Risk Assessment

Are you at risk for fracture? The answer is yes, if you have osteoporosis, osteopoenia, or low bone density. Do you know what movements and activities put you at a high risk for fracture? Check the boxes next to the everyday activity questions to which you would answer yes. Then see how you did at the end of the test. (This quiz is intended for you only if you have been diagnosed with osteoporosis or osteopoenia.)

- ❏ Do you bend over to tie your shoes?

- ❏ Do you stand or sit with poor posture?

- ❏ Do you walk with your feet pointed out to the sides?

- ❏ Do you bend over when you mop, sweep, or vacuum, to get to those hard to reach places?

- ❏ Do you bend over to pick things up off the floor?

- ❏ Does your torso jolt forward when you sneeze or cough?

- ❏ Do you sit straight up, without rolling to one side first, when you get out of bed?

- ❏ Do you walk on icy, wet, or slippery surfaces?

☐ Do you do sit-ups on the floor or with exercise equipment?

☐ Do you do step aerobics?

☐ Do you do kick boxing?

☐ Do you perform abdominal exercises on machines or on the floor that have you twist from side to side?

☐ Do you perform any leg exercises that make your legs go to the sides of your body?

☐ Do you take spinning classes or go bike riding with your chest bent forward over the handlebars?

☐ Do you wear flip-flops or slippers that are open behind your heel?

☐ Is your favorite chair one that allows you to sink into it?

☐ Do you play golf?

☐ Do you ice-skate?

☐ Do you downhill ski?

☐ Do you reach for objects off of high shelves?

☐ Do you play tennis without turning your entire body to hit a backhand stroke?

☐ Do you spend a lot of time in bed (other than the 8–10 hours for sleeping each night)?

☐ Do you lift objects or babies weighing more than 10 pounds?

☐ Do you lean forward so that your head and shoulders are over your knees when you get out of a chair?

**If you checked one or more of the boxes above, you are at high risk for a fracture!**

All of the situations listed above are potentially dangerous for someone with low bone density. By the time you finish reading this chapter, you will have learned to modify these activities so that you can do many of them safely, without risk of fracture. You'll also find that some of the activities listed are impossible to modify in order to make them safe for someone with low bone density. By the end of the chapter you'll have a strong understanding of what makes any movement safe or potentially dangerous for someone with low bone density.

# The 5 Golden Rules for Avoiding Fracture

Have you ever been a little pregnant? No, me either. In fact, I was a big, fat pregnant hog. Well, the same goes for osteoporosis. You cannot have just a "little" osteoporosis. If you have been diagnosed with osteoporosis, you have been diagnosed with "severe and advanced low bone density." **These rules apply to you!** A study by the International Osteoporosis Foundation has uncovered the emotional and physical effects that osteoporosis has on women living with the disease. The study revealed that 37 percent of women with osteoporosis suffered from back pain, 30 percent were constantly afraid that they would break a bone, 29 percent were unable to walk long distances, and 18 percent expressed difficulty just getting from point A to point B. Additionally, 17 percent were worried about their futures—how long would they be independent? Overall, 81 percent recognized that the disease had affected them adversely. You can gain relief from many of these concerns just by knowing how to avoid fracture—how to stay safe.

These "5 Golden Rules" of osteoporosis were my motivation for writing this book. Many doctors have sent me their osteoporosis patients to help them increase bone density. However, *not one* of those clients has been familiar with the following postures that need to be avoided in order to reduce their risk of bone fracture. You *must* be informed about what increases the risk of fracture, and you *must* apply this knowledge to your everyday life and your exercise program. You are taking charge of your condition by reading this book. Be sure to make it effective by becoming familiar with the following fracture-risk postures. Not only will you lower your risk of a broken bone, but your exercise program will be a success.

Did you know that most fractures happen in the home, during the late afternoon? This tidbit of information tells us that fractures are not necessarily happening during a step aerobics class or while grocery shopping, but during that sleepy time of day in the late afternoon when our senses are a bit dulled and our coordination is not quite at peak levels. The 5 Golden Rules will help you to reduce your fracture risk, regardless of what you may be doing.

## Golden Rule #1:
## Do Not Flex the Spine!

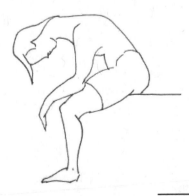

This rule is for anyone with osteoporosis of the spine, which includes the neck. Flexing the spine is simply bending forward at the waist or dropping the head forward (chin to chest). This is the type of movement typical of reaching for something on the floor while seated or performing a sit-up. No more sit-ups! You do not have to perform "crunches" or sit-ups to strengthen the abdominals (I'll tell you how in just a moment).

There are many times during the course of the day when it is natural for us to flex the spine. Flexing the spine can include activities such as putting on your shoes, mopping the floor, carrying groceries, picking items up off the floor, or even laying down in bed. You must modify all of these activities by keeping your spine straight. Do not allow your shoulders to sink forward, pulling the spine down. The following are some common activities during which mistakes are frequently made. Get to know them, and apply this first rule to all of your activities.

### Picking Items Up Off the Ground

Whatever it is, we all frequently have to retrieve something that has fallen to the floor. If you are as unfortunate as I am to have a dog that relishes chewing up all the junk mail *every* afternoon when the mailman arrives, then you are on the floor quite a bit. When you want to pick something up that is on the floor, be sure to begin with a straight spine. Kneel down on one knee and then the other. If there is a wall or a couch nearby, you can use that for support as you lower yourself to the floor. If you have a lot of work to do while you are down there, such as scrubbing a bathtub, gardening, or picking up microscopic pieces of torn junk mail, position yourself on your hands and knees. Keep your shoulders back and do not bend forward at the waist or slouch the shoulders forward as you work.

To tie your shoes or paint your toenails, first prop up your foot on a stool in front of you. Now you can more easily reach your feet without having to bend the spine. Keep your spine straight.

**Yes!**            **No**

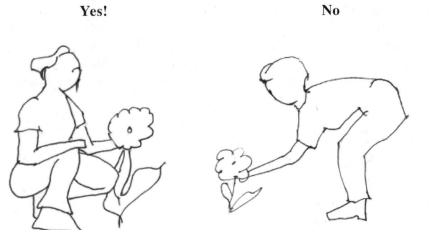

## Pushing a Carriage, a Broom, a Vacuum Cleaner, or Anything at All

To push a carriage, mop the floor, vacuum a rug, or rake leaves, always maintain a straight spine. Do not reach forward so that you are bending at the waist. Keep an eye on your shoulders for cues to your posture. If your shoulders are rounded, there is a good chance that you are not working with a straight spine. Keep your spine straight.

**Yes!** **No**

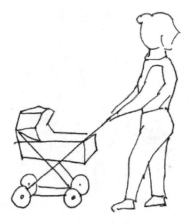 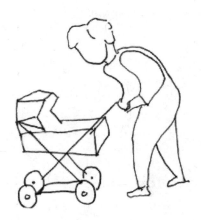

## Exercise Class

In exercise classes, you will be met with many challenges, especially when it comes to working on abdominal exercises. No more sit-ups! Sit-ups put you in a *very* high fracture-risk situation. Not only are you flexing the spine, but the weight of your torso, along with the force of gravity, puts a tremendous amount of pressure on your vertebrae. I have worked with people with osteopoenia (which is low bone density, but not as severe as osteoporosis) who have found out that they had low bone density because of small fractures that were a result of an abdominal class at the local gym. If someone with osteopoenia can fracture her spine doing sit-ups and crunches, someone with osteoporosis is certainly going to want to avoid those exercises. You'll have to be sure not to bend the spine forward during any part of your workout. You'll find that many of the exercises in the following chapters have modifications that you can apply in your exercise classes.

**No More Sit-ups!**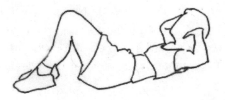

### An Alternative Abdominal Exercise

The abdominal exercise below is very safe and *extremely* effective. I give this exercise to all of my clients, low bone density or not. I like it because it really works, and it challenges people regardless of their fitness level. It also forces people to work their abdominal muscles correctly, creating a flat tummy instead of thick abdominal muscles which can look like a layer of fat.

### Alternative Abdominal Exercise

**Flat Spine!**                **Move from the hip—knees stay bent.**

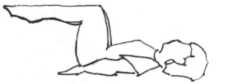 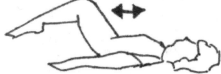

### How It's Done

Lie flat on your back and bring your feet off the floor so that your knees are directly over your hips and your lower legs are parallel to the ground. Now, instead of crunching and bringing the shoulders up and down (that would be flexing the spine), you are going to press your thighs away from you until you feel tension in your stomach. Be sure to make the movement happen at the hip. The knees do not straighten or bend—they stay at the same 90-degree angle the whole time. You should only be able to move the thighs away from you a couple of inches if your spine is truly pressed down on the mat. Cheating does not help you to tone and gain strength. Now bring your thighs back toward you again. Just repeat this while the rest of the class is doing their sit-ups. You'll be keeping your spine safe while performing a very challenging and effective abdominal exercise—and your classmates will be jealous because your stomach will actually be getting flatter.

**Abdominal exercise alert! Do them wrong and your stomach gets bigger!** No more "poochy" tummies. When you work on your abdominal muscles, your abdominals must remain *flat*—not poochy. Poochy is that look you get when the stomach muscles bulge when they are working. If your muscles bulge when working, that is the shape you will be forming. Your stomach will actually get bigger, not smaller.

Are you doing your abdominal work incorrectly? I can only tell you that I have never had a new client do abdominal work correctly. What does that mean? It means that most of the people at the gym are getting bigger stomachs, hence all the frustration you hear from people hammering away at their abdominals at the gym. I actually had two women taking Pilates with me and doing abdominal classes at the gym. They were on a mission for flatter stomachs. Both women had bigger waists by the end of the month. Their stomachs were actually growing instead of diminishing. Once they incorporated what I had shown them about keeping the stomach flat, their pants began to fit again. Do the abdominal exercise described above with your stomach muscles flat and you'll not only be getting stronger, but chances are you'll be the only one in class not getting a "poochy tummy."

### Carrying Groceries and Children

When you carry groceries, do not allow the weight of the bags to pull your spine forward. The general recommendation is to carry weights of 10 pounds or less, so you'll want to be sure to pack light and possibly make more trips back-and-forth to the car. Again, while carrying and lifting, maintain a straight, neutral spine. Because most children weigh more than 10 pounds, have them crawl onto your lap once you are already sitting. Be sure to inform any grandchildren that jumping off the middle of the stairs and into your arms is going to be out of the question from now on.

### Lying Down on Your Exercise Mat

Lying down on your exercise mat or getting out of bed in the morning can be a lot like performing a sit-up, depending on how you do it. Getting on and off the floor by rolling through your stomach puts a tremendous amount of pressure on your vertebrae because of the combined force of gravity and your body weight. To lower yourself to the floor, try this instead: While keeping your back straight, first kneel on one knee and then the other. Lower your hips to one side of your feet and continue lowering yourself onto your side. Now, just roll onto your back.

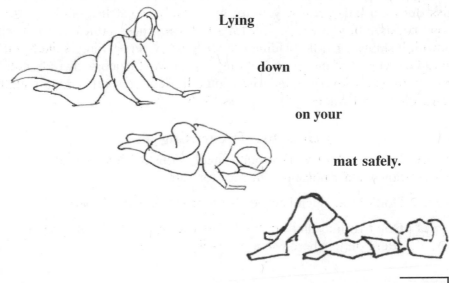

**Lying down on your mat safely.**

### Allergies and Colds

Having experienced two herniated disks, I know how much pressure coughing and sneezing puts on the spine. It's a tremendous amount of pressure, much more than any sit-up. In fact, you probably know someone with healthy bone density who has cracked a rib from coughing when they had a particularly bad cold.

One of the hardest moments to maintain proper posture and to avoid flexing the spine is during coughing and sneezing. You want to do whatever you can to maintain a straight spine when you must cough or if you feel a sneeze coming on. Press your spine into the back of a chair or the wall, and try to keep it there. When my back was bad, I used to grab the arms of the chair in order to keep my spine from bending. Be careful—you can usually feel a sneeze coming on, so be prepared.

## Golden Rule #2: Do Not Put Excessive Pressure on the Wrists

If you have osteoporosis at either wrist, or if you have not been tested for osteoporosis at the wrist but have osteoporosis of the spine, you will

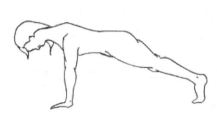

want to avoid putting harmful pressure on the wrist joint. I tell my clients that if they have tested positively for osteoporosis of the spine, the likelihood of the wrist having low bone density is high. The wrist, similar to the spine because of the high percentage of spongy bone, is susceptible to loss of bone mass. While the wrist bones can be in jeopardy during certain sports like tennis, baseball, or just doing a push-up, if your bone loss is severe, the wrist bones are at their highest risk during a fall. Because you are most likely to catch a fall by putting your hands out, you are at risk for shattering these bones. Ice-skating, downhill skiing, or rollerblading are all sports where falling is likely—it's an expected part of the sport. Not only is your wrist in jeopardy of fracture, but so are your hip and spine when you fall. Begin researching an equally rewarding sport where spills are less likely.

### Don'ts for Preventing Falls

❑ Don't walk or work around highly polished floors—put down some nonslip area rugs for safety.

❑ Don't wear open-backed shoes or shoes with slippery soles.

❑ Don't rush around so much that you may not be able to pay attention to where you are stepping.

- ❑ Don't walk on icy surfaces that haven't been salted or sanded.

- ❑ Don't participate in activities where falling is probable, such as ice-skating, rollerblading, and downhill skiing.

- ❑ Don't keep rugs in your home that slide around or fold up in the corners—secure them or get rid of them.

- ❑ Don't keep your pet's water where it may spill and cause a fall.

- ❑ Don't carry large loads (even if they are light) that prevent you from seeing where you are stepping.

- ❑ Don't stand on a chair to reach a top shelf—buy a stepladder with railings.

- ❑ Don't walk with poor posture—you won't be able to see where you are going if you are bent over.

- ❑ Don't allow pets to get underfoot when you are busy doing tasks, such as working in the kitchen.

## Do's for Preventing Falls

- ❑ Do perform a regular exercise program (such as the three available in Chapter 6) that improves strength, balance, flexibility, and coordination. A strong body can be your best defense against a fall. Studies have shown that seniors, out of any age group, have the most to gain from an exercise program. The good news is that, as a senior, your ability to increase strength has not changed since you were a teenager.

- ❑ Do keep the 5 Golden Rules in mind, these guidelines can greatly reduce your fall risk by keeping you in proper alignment at all times.

- ❑ Do regular checks in your home for loose carpets, and decaying or loose boards on stairs or outdoor steps.

- ❑ Do place double-sided tape or antislip rubber mats under your rugs.

- ❑ Do be extremely cautious on any tiled surfaces in your home. You may want to place rugs with an antislip rubber mat in these places, in case of a water spill that can make the floor extremely slippery.

- ❑ Do place rubber mats or handrails in the shower.

- ❑ Do use the handrail when climbing steps. Using the handrail also prevents you from carrying too much when going up and down stairs, which can also cause a fall.

❑ Do remain active and enjoy yourself. Do not allow the fact that you have osteoporosis to scare you away from your activities. An active life will add to your ability to build bone density. Sitting at home is the worst possible alternative, because long periods of immobility will reduce your bone density. Besides that, it is just plain depressing to be cooped up.

## A Special Note About Osteoporosis at the Wrist

Because bone becomes denser in direct response to force from the muscles, when you are beginning to build your bone density at the wrist, just like anywhere else, you have to start easy and build up to harder exercises. Changes in bone density will only occur if you are progressively challenging the muscles, which in turn progressively ask more of the bone. As the bone tissue responds to the extra muscular work with thicker bone, you will be able to try more difficult exercises or tasks. However, be sure to stay in touch with your doctor to see how the bone density is progressing before you try a new sport, such as tennis. As an interesting note, tennis players are generally not at risk for osteoporosis at the wrist of the arm with which they hold their racket because bone becomes denser where force is applied to the muscles. Tennis players have strong arms and forearms and, therefore, denser bone mass at the wrist.

## Create a Strong Core to Prevent Falling

Your core muscles are your deep abdominal and spine muscles. The core muscles are crucial when it comes to preventing a fall, thus protecting the wrists. We all know that feeling of slipping and knowing we can either "catch" ourselves or fall to the floor. The core muscles are the "catching" muscles. They help us maintain our balance. Working on these muscles with the OsteoPilates programs at the end of Chapter 6 will give you more strength in your core and more ability to balance and prevent falls.

## Golden Rule #3: Do Not Abduct Your Legs

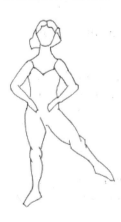

This is especially important for someone with osteoporosis of the hip or someone with osteoporosis of the spine who has not had the bone density at the hip checked. To lower your risk of hip fracture, do not abduct or carry your legs to the sides and away from the center of your body. You can take your leg straight in front of you or straight back without risk of a hip fracture but not out to the sides of your body. Leg abduction is found in many exercises, martial arts, and dance classes. If you participate in any of these activities you'll want to modify your movement at that point in the class.

## A Note About Skiing

I know from personal experience that many of my crash-landings on the ski slopes have put me in a position of very painful leg abduction (an acrobatic split, for example, with my hips killing me and my skis far from straight under me). Skiing, especially downhill, is probably a sport you want to think long and hard about returning to because of the high fracture-risk possibilities that it presents. Have you ever been snowshoeing? It's a blast! It's a great workout, and snowshoeing is usually done on some quiet, pristine mountaintop far from the maddening crowds of ski slopes. Also, I have never been run over by an errant snowshoer who is snowshoeing out of control behind me.

## Walking

Part of not abducting the legs is not turning the feet out when you walk. Be sure to point your feet directly ahead (like railroad tracks) when you walk. Walking with your feet straight ahead is proper body mechanics. For someone with osteoporosis, walking with the feet pointed directly ahead will reduce the risk of tripping and falling. When you begin snowshoeing, you'll be able to tell exactly where your feet are pointing—just look at your tracks. Of course, you could also inspect your footprints as you take a stroll along the beach.

**Yes!** **No**

# Golden Rule #4:
# Do Not Twist the Spine

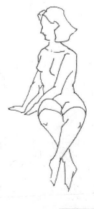

Twisting the spine is a very high fracture-risk situation for those with osteoporosis of the spine. Situations of twisting with force, such as playing tennis, golfing, or reaching for groceries in the backseat while sitting in the frontseat, are all dangerous fracture situations. If you attend a local gym, you may have noticed that there is gym equipment specifically designed for gaining strength while twisting the spine. Avoid not only those machines but any exercise that twists the spine.

## The Top Shelf

If you are reaching for something that is on a top shelf, be careful not to twist the spine as you stretch for that item. Generally, when we reach with just one hand, it is because we are trying to gain extra length or height by twisting the spine. Instead, reach with both arms to avoid twisting the spine. If you still cannot reach your item, you may want to use a stepladder with handrails to put yourself up high enough to easily reach the item.

**Yes!**                                                      **No**

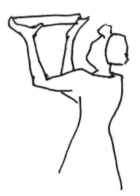 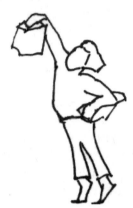

## Twisting Abdominal Exercises

This common abdominal exercise is to be avoided. This exercise breaks Golden Rule #1: *Do not flex the spine* and Golden Rule #4: *Do not twist the spine*. If you are participating in an exercise class where this is being taught, do the modified abdominal exercise shown in the "Do Not Flex the Spine" section of this chapter on page 58.

**No**

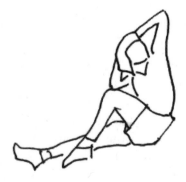

## Golden Rule #5: Do Not Sit or Stand With Poor Posture

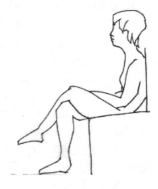

Everyone I have ever met is sick of hearing about how poor their posture is. Chances are you aren't thrilled about a potential lecture on perfect posture either, but bear with me. Attaining improved posture is easier than you have previously been led to believe—I promise. First things first, though. Why is poor posture dangerous to someone with osteoporosis? Will the benefits of improved posture be worth the effort?

Yes, avoid sitting or standing with poor posture and you will reduce your risk of fracture at all sites of osteoporosis. The flexed spine position of poor posture puts more pressure on the vertebrae, making them more likely to fracture (see Golden Rule #1 on page 55). Poor posture also makes falling more likely, resulting in hip and wrist fractures.

There are more benefits to standing up straight than just avoiding a fracture. Applying good postural habits will create more strength and flexibility in your abdominals and spine. This increased strength will improve your balance and help with coordination and ease of movement in everyday activities. You'll feel better! And after all, isn't that the goal in all of this?

### Good Posture for the Yogi in You

Because yoga is the direct ancestor of Pilates exercise, it will be beneficial for us to take a moment to see what yoga has to say about good posture. Yogis teach us that there are seven *chakras* or energy centers. They begin at the base of your spine and lead to the crown of your head. Proper posture opens up these chakras and allows the life force to flow through you. Poor posture clogs up your energy. When energy does not flow, you will feel tired and you will be more likely to succumb to disease, stress, or depression.

### Shoulder, Back, and Neck Pain With Poor Posture

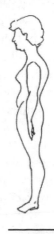

This drawing represents a very common example of poor posture. This woman is doing a lot of extra work just to remain vertical. The extra work that her muscles are constantly required to do creates aches and pains that most people believe are common with aging. They are not. They are aches and pains that are common with poor posture at *all* ages.

Starting from the top, her upper back is rounded, which naturally causes her head to drop forward. To hold her head up, she has to recruit extra muscles in the back of her neck and shoulders, forcing those muscles to work overtime, which leads to achy neck and upper back muscles. The shoulders are tight and rounded, indicated by the palms of her hands facing behind her (relaxed arms should have palms facing the thighs). Her poor shoulder alignment adds to the problem of her rounded upper back and, again, over-recruits the muscles in neck and upper back.

Her poor upper back posture would make it very difficult to stand up at all if it weren't for her hips protruding too far forward in order to compensate for the poor posture and to keep her balanced. In this postural position it is very difficult for her to engage or use her stomach muscles at all. As a result, they are completely relaxed, which makes it appear that she has a little bit of a "tummy" on her. In reality though, the woman in this drawing is plenty thin and, if she was able to stand up straight, her "tummy" would disappear. The protrusion of the relaxed stomach muscles has also resulted in locked knees, which lead to knee pain. Overall, this woman could use some postural improvement techniques because she is undoubtedly in pain.

You may know someone who looks like the woman in the drawing—it's really not uncommon. Go to the mall and you will definitely find several people that look like this drawing. You will also find many other variations of imperfect alignment. People get caught in some very bad postural habits that can result in years of pain and discomfort. If they only knew… But not you. Keep reading and you'll find out how to improve your posture and your health.

## A Quick Note About Breathing and Posture

Breathing patterns are also improved with proper posture. Your lungs won't be pressed or collapsed upon, and your new breathing patterns (also see the "Breathing" exercise on page 123) may decrease low back, shoulder, and neck pain, according to a study from the American Physiological Society, conducted by P. Hodges, S. Gandevia, and C. Richardson. Lower fracture risk, better energy flow for improved health and better breathing patterns for reduced pain—improved posture is looking pretty darn good!

## Standing and Sitting With Correct Posture

We've all had parents or friends tell us to "Stand up straight!" or "Don't slouch!" I certainly have memories of my mother telling me, or of her walking up behind me and yanking my shoulders back into a *straight* position. Sound familiar? But what does it really mean to stand and sit with good posture or correct alignment? You'll be happy to learn that the shoulders yanked way back behind your ears is *not* correct alignment. That is a misalignment, often referred to as military stance, where the chest sticks out in front, the chin is pulled in, and shoulder blades are aggressively pinching together. When I ask my clients to stand with correct posture, military stance is usually what I get. Correct posture is actually much simpler than that. Situate yourself next to a mirror, bring this book along, and you'll see how easy it is to find correct alignment.

## How to Stand Up Straight

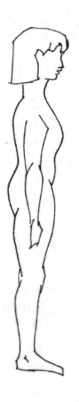

Begin by standing with your side facing a full-length mirror.

- Imagine that someone is pulling a single strand of your hair up to the ceiling. That single hair is going to lengthen your spine up just like a puppet on a string.

- As you glance sideways into the mirror, your ear should be in line with your shoulder.

- An imaginary line from your shoulder should drop through the middle of your hip.

- This same line should drop to your knee, on the back of your leg.

- From your knee, the line should drop through the middle of the ankle.

- While in correct alignment, there should be a natural curve at your lower back and behind your neck. Your palms should face your thighs, indicating adequate flexibility at the shoulders.

## The Test

Now back up against a wall with your heels approximately 2–3 inches from the wall. You should feel the back of your head, your upper back, and your hips touching the wall. Do not push your head against the wall by lifting the chin and looking up at the ceiling (that would be cheating). Tuck the chin and pull it back toward your throat.

## Rounded Upper Back

What if you have lined your spine up properly according to the previous advice, but when you back up to the wall, you can only get your upper back and hips to touch the wall and not your head (regardless of how much you pull your chin in)? Depending on age and determination, this posture may be less easy to fix than the rounded shoulders. I do encourage you to try to do everything you can to change it, though. A rounded upper back with osteoporosis violates Golden Rule #1: Do Not Flex the Spine, and you should work at changing that posture everyday. More likely than not, a rounded upper back has probably resulted in neck and shoulder pain for you. The more you work to reduce the roundness in your upper back, the better your neck and shoulders are going to feel because they won't be fighting against the pressures of incorrect posture.

### Did You Know?

Just because someone may have a rounded upper back does not mean he or she has osteoporosis. I have worked with many clients with osteoporosis who have had extremely wonderful posture. I have also worked with the opposite—a severely rounded upper back without osteoporosis.

### What You Can Do Today for a Rounded Upper Back

First, start with the beginning OsteoPilates program at the end of Chapter 7 on page 177. The exercises in this program directly address the issues of osteoporosis and focus on strengthening the upper back, which facilitates good posture and a less rounded spine.

However, without going on to the exercises at the end of Chapter 7, there are two things that you can start doing *right now*:

- *Gently* pinch your shoulder blades together. This one simple exercise will begin to strengthen the muscles in your upper back and allow any tightness at the front of the shoulders to begin releasing. You can do this during all of your waking hours, whether you are sitting, standing, kneeling, driving, or doing any activity at all.

- Perform the "Football Shoulders" exercise explained on page 69. Do it a few times a day to reinforce proper positioning of your shoulders.

### Rounded Shoulders

What if you have lined everything up properly but your shoulders are curling forward? That is a muscular imbalance. It is actually quite common with humans. All of our work is done in front of us with our arms forward—driving, cooking, lifting, gardening, etc. The muscles at the front of your shoulders are stronger and less flexible than the muscles at the back of the shoulders.

There is a shoulder stretch and many shoulder exercises in Chapter 7 that address this imbalance. We will be working on getting the muscles between the shoulder blades as strong, if not stronger, than the muscles at the front of the shoulders, as well as stretching the fronts of the shoulders so that the stronger muscles that we are building in your upper back will be able to pull the shoulders back, and they won't be fighting against tight muscles. After all, if those muscles can be made so strong to throw you out of alignment doesn't it make sense that we can reverse that imbalance so that the muscles between the shoulder blades naturally pull us to a position of proper alignment? It does make sense, and it is very possible. I have worked with many clients with shoulder "issues," and they tell me that their posture at their computers has improved dramatically within a few weeks. They also tell me that it has become uncomfortable for them to sit with poor posture. See? It's possible.

## Think "Football Shoulders"

This is an image I often give to my clients and, no, your shoulders won't get big—it's just an image. Standing or sitting up straight, put your arms directly out to your sides so that they are parallel to the ground. Now, imagine that your shoulders extend all the way out to your fingertips. Slowly, lower your arms, but keep the image that your shoulders are still out by your fingertips. Your shoulders should feel wide and not pinched together. I always feel long and stretched across the front of my shoulders when I do this exercise. It feels great! It feels like the front of my chest has been released and opened. Do this exercise several times a day to correct the position of your shoulders. Before you know it you'll perform "Football Shoulders" and nothing will change because your shoulders are already properly placed.

## Good Posture... It's Not Just About Standing up Straight

As you know from Golden Rule #1, the spine should not flex forward. Maintaining good posture is not just about looking taller, younger, and more alert, it is about not creating a fracture-risk situation. When your spine is bent forward and not lengthening to the ceiling, it is supporting a lot of extra weight that it should not be supporting. Not only is your spine supporting the weight of your upper body (chest, shoulders, arms, neck, and head), it is constantly working against gravity. Imagine a building on which the top third of its architecture is bent forward. Eventually, it is going to break. The strongest beams cannot work against weight and gravity day in and day out—and neither can your spine.

## Marshmallows and the Dowager's Hump

If the spine fractures, it is usually on the front of the spine, or the part facing the stomach. With each little fracture, the spine collapses forward. Imagine pinching a whole column of marshmallows on one side. You would be creating a replica of the dowager's hump that is often associated with osteoporosis. Sometimes this hump is just due to decades of poor posture. Don't assume that because you or a friend has a rounded upper back that it is a result of vertebral fractures.

## Correlation Between Height Loss and Vertebral Fracture

Many people with a vertebral fracture do not know that they have experienced a fracture. Doctors at the University of Alberta, Edmonton have found a correlation between height loss and vertebral fracture that may help you to know if you have actually experienced a fracture without even knowing it. If you have lost two centimeters of height over the past three years, there is a significant possibility that you have experienced a vertebral fracture.

## A Postural Mystery

Standing up straight *is* a mystery for most people. Good posture is often equated with being uncomfortable and unhappy. That is *not* what you should be feeling. Standing up straight should feel like the easiest way to stand because it takes the most possible pressure off of your spine; your vertebrae are aligned in an erect position, minimizing the effects of gravity and the weight of your upper body.

## Building Blocks to Spinal Success

Just like a child's building blocks, your spine will be most able to sustain an upright position if the vertebrae are stacked one on top of the other. Only their natural curve should take them away from a perfectly straight spine. This balanced position takes mechanical stress off of your spine and therefore off of your shoulders, neck, and hips. Because all body parts lead back to the spine, any imbalance in the alignment of the back will cause imbalances elsewhere, usually resulting in chronic pain. Clients I see who have chronic neck and shoulder pain are addressed for their postural misalignments first. Many report pain relief after their first class. It's not magic. A body that is put back into alignment is naturally going to be more pain free.

## Sitting With Good Posture

*Sitting* with good posture and proper alignment is easy once you clearly understand the previous elements for *standing* up straight. Many of the same rules apply.

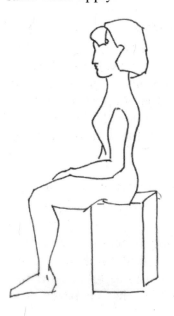

- Imagine a single strand of your hair is being pulled up to the ceiling. This single strand lengthens your spine from your hips to the top of your head.

- An imaginary line should pass through your ear, to the middle of your shoulder, to the middle of your hip.

- If you can position your knees slightly below your hips, this will help to tilt your hips forward and prevent slumping into the low back.

## Choosing a Chair

If you sit in a soft chair, it is going to be extremely difficult to maintain proper alignment while seated. A firm chair will give you the support you need to maintain proper alignment of the spine. A soft chair is going to make it very difficult for you to avoid flexing your spine (Golden Rule #1).

### Golden Rule Reminder Chart

**#1 Do not flex the spine!**
Regardless of your activity, you should never bend forward from the waist.

**#2 Do not put excessive pressure on the wrists.**
The wrist joint can only take so much, and when it breaks, it is generally a multiple fracture.

**#3 Do not abduct the legs.**
Keep your legs going straight ahead of you or behind you, and avoid allowing them to travel out to the sides of your body.

**#4 Do not twist the spine.**
Avoid rotating from your waist. Move your spine as one solid piece.

**#5 Do not stand or sit with poor posture.**
The hardest one of all, perfect posture will not only prevent fracture, but it will also create strength and better health.

# Review, Review, and Review Again

All of the advice in this chapter may seem quite overwhelming. There is, without a doubt, quite a lot to absorb. Go ahead and read and reread until the information seems commonplace and you have been able to apply the 5 Golden Rules for avoiding fracture, as well as the advice for maintaining proper alignment. But even if you don't feel like you have grasped all of the information (check your knowledge on the "List of Understanding" that follows), do continue to read further. Just come back to this chapter for review as often as possible, until everything feels second nature to you. It is not impossible to have perfect posture. You *can* do it, and you *will* do it. Even though you may not have perfect posture overnight, it is very likely that you will start feeling better almost immediately. Be sure to be gentle with yourself and take the time to take small steps forward. Steps that are too big usually result in giving up altogether.

## List of Understanding

When these following points begin to make sense, you'll know you have grasped the key points of this chapter.

- The 5 Golden Rules of avoiding fractures.

- Correct posture vs. military stance.

- Football shoulders vs. rounded shoulders.

- An alternative abdominal activity for exercise class.

- What you can do today for a rounded upper back.

# Chapter 4

## The Milkshake Diet: *Nutrition for Osteoporosis*

Moving right along, we come to the second part of your four-part plan. Proper nutrition for osteoporosis is probably the easiest and most enjoyable component to implement into your better bone plan. Studies have shown that exercise programs and medications, too, become much more effective for increasing bone density when added to a healthy diet that is high in calcium. Remember that all of the components of an osteoporosis plan—exercise, medication, postural awareness, and diet—have a greater combined effect than any one component by itself. In other words, the sum is greater than all the parts. In fact, some studies have shown diet to be completely ineffective on its own but that it greatly increases the effectiveness of an exercise program when the two are used together.

Because this chapter does not discuss dieting to lose weight (most people with osteoporosis are quite thin anyway—even if they don't think so), the changes we will be making in this chapter are to include foods that taste great but also have an adequate amount of calcium and vitamin D for promoting bone growth. So think of this as the "Milkshake Diet" not the "Rabbit Food Diet."

Having another milkshake isn't always the answer, though. Some people are religiously getting enough calcium in their diets, but their bodies are not absorbing it. We'll be looking at factors that may be hindering your ability to absorb calcium and discuss how to improve absorption. Sometimes the problem is easy to fix; it could be that the supplement you are taking is not dissolving—I'll show you a trick for finding out if it is. After you know that you are absorbing calcium, there are diet plans and some great recipes to help you boost calcium in your diet. But first, let's start with how much calcium you need in the first place.

# Calcium

Are you getting enough? Chances are that you are not, according to national nutrition surveys. These surveys have shown that Caucasian, Hispanic, and African-American women all consume less than half the amount of calcium suggested for healthy bone growth. Asian women consume 50 percent more than their Western counterparts do.

## Recommended Calcium Intake in the United States

The following chart includes all age groups because it is believed that low calcium intake throughout life is responsible for low bone density and high fracture rate later in life. The second chart, from the National Institute of Health, is great because it differentiates between how much calcium a postmenopausal woman on estrogen needs, as opposed to a postmenopausal woman who is not on estrogen.

| Age | Recommended Daily Intake |
| --- | --- |
| Birth to 3 years | 400–800 mg, 1–2 cups of milk |
| 4–10 years | 800–1200 mg, 2–3 cups of milk |
| Adolescent and Adult Males | 800–1200 mg, 2–3 cups of milk |
| Adolescent and Adult Females | 800–1200 mg, 2–3 cups of milk |
| Pregnant Females | 1200 mg, 3 cups of milk |
| Breast-feeding Females | 1200 mg, 3 cups of milk |

### Calcium Recommendations for Women Over 50

| | |
| --- | --- |
| Women over 50, Postmenopausal, taking estrogen | 1,000 mg/day |
| Women over 50, Postmenopausal, not taking estrogen | 1,500 mg/day |

*Source: National Institute of Health

## 400 Mg of Calcium Every Day! Or Is It 800 Mg?

You may have already noticed that, where some vitamins or minerals are concerned, there seems to be quite a bit of distance between the low end and the high end of the recommended daily intake. The broad range of possibilities seems almost absurd. After all, if I asked my son how many kids were at the party he went to last weekend, I wouldn't expect him to say, "2 or 22, I'm not really sure, Mom." Such large ranges of possibility aren't generally applied in our lives, so why here, where our nutritional well-being is at stake?

Unfortunately, this large range for a recommended daily allowance reflects the uncertainty of the science of regulating vitamins and minerals. Regulation becomes difficult because scientists are trying to create an average number that will be beneficial to the average person. For the reader of this book, who is probably more active than the average person, your dietary allowance might be different than a sedentary person.

Or what about a person with a chronic disease? Do they need different dietary guidelines, also? That sort of information is exactly what the National Academy of Sciences is trying to discern. The National Academy of Sciences regularly publishes updates to their list of dietary allowances, and the lists are hopefully more and more accurate each time. In other words, the recommendations you see here are the very best that science has to offer. But don't be surprised when you look at the requirement for a certain vitamin or mineral and see a big gap between the high end and low end of what is considered to be the recommended daily allowance. And don't be surprised if new research significantly changes these recommendations in the future.

## Eating! The Fun Way to Get Your Calcium

Calcium doesn't come only in supplements. Our cave ancestors certainly weren't running down to the local cave/vitamin store to order calcium tablets from their local supplement guru/Neanderthal—although, it makes for an interesting image. We can, however, learn from our Neanderthal friends and procure our necessary nutrients from food. The list on page 76 should help you get going in the right direction.

## The Difference Between Consumption and Absorption

Many of you are already concerned with bone density and probably are doing your best to boost your daily calcium intake with supplements and dietary changes. For many people, though, there is a big difference between what we digest and what our bodies are absorbing. The reasons vary. It could be that the vitamin you are taking is not absorbable, or perhaps you are lactose intolerant. Current research reveals that there may even be a connection between calcium absorption and high protein intake.

## The Vitamin Disintegration Test

If your calcium supplement doesn't disintegrate, then the calcium won't be absorbed into your bloodstream, which in turn won't be able to deliver adequate calcium supplies to the bones. That fact seems blatantly obvious,

| Food | Milligrams of Calcium |
|---|---|
| Almonds (2 oz.) | 150 |
| American Cheese (1 oz.) | 174 |
| Broccoli (frozen, 1/2 cup) | 50 |
| Cheddar Cheese (1 oz.) | 204 |
| Collards (1/2 cup) | 70 |
| Cottage Cheese—lowfat (1 cup) | 154 |
| Ice Cream  (3/4 cup) | 120 |
| Ice Cream—Soft Serve (3/4 cup) | 205 |
| Ice Milk (3/4 cup) | 132 |
| Milk—lowfat, skim, or whole (1 cup)    Hint: The lower the fat,    the higher the calcium. | 275-400 |
| Mozzarella—part skim (2 oz.) | 300 |
| Orange Juice with Calcium (1 cup) | 400 |
| Oysters—raw (6 oysters) | 36 |
| Ricotta Cheese, part skim (1/2 cup) | 340 |
| Salmon—canned with bones (2 oz.) | 120 |
| Shrimp (1 cup) | 147 |
| Soybeans (1/2 cup) | 89 |
| Swiss Cheese (1 oz.) | 272 |
| Tofu (1/2 cup) | 125 |

but how many of us have ever tested our vitamins for disintegration? I know I never did until I ran across this great tip. Just drop one of your calcium tablets into about 2/3 cup of vinegar or warm water and stir once in a while. In 30 minutes, the tablet should have disintegrated. If it did not, you may want to try another brand name or a calcium compound tablet such as calcium carbonate and calcium citrate together. Calcium supplements are generally more easily absorbed when taken in small doses throughout the day and with food.

A recent study at Creighton University revealed that only 2 out of 8 calcium carbonate supplements are as absorbable as plain calcium carbonate that has not been put into a pill form. Once calcium carbonate has been taken from its purest form and manufacturing processes have added coatings and flavorings, the milligrams of calcium that become available decreases considerably. Check your own tablets using the disintegration test to see if they will be absorbed or stay whole in your stomach.

## Lactose Intolerance

Lactose intolerance, or the inability to digest dairy products, affects approximately 40 million Americans. Their inability to break down milk sugars, also called lactose, prevents these individuals from being able to absorb calcium from the milk products they consume. According to the National Institute of Diabetes and Digestive and Kidney Diseases (NIDDK), 75 percent of adult African-Americans and Native Americans and 90 percent of Asian-Americans are unable to digest lactose. Because consuming dairy products results in gas, cramps, and diarrhea in those who are lactose intolerant, it is understandable that they stay away from anything with milk content. Although, even if they were to consume dairy products, they would not be able to absorb the calcium offered there. This puts them at high risk for developing osteoporosis.

Some people who are lactose intolerant are still able to tolerate some dairy products divided into small servings throughout the day, while others develop symptoms with even the smallest amount of milk (or whey) found in store-bought bread. There are alternatives, though. First, there are dairy products that contain lactase, the enzyme necessary for digesting milk products. This added lactase can make milk products entirely digestible for those who would otherwise become sick with stomach cramps and possibly vomiting from their inability to break down the lactose (milk sugars) in dairy products. Yogurt with active cultures is also an option for some lactose intolerant people.

There are, of course, alternatives to drinking milk or consuming dairy products. Refer back to the previous list (page 76) for foods that are high in calcium.

## Protein and Good Diet Linked With Better Calcium Absorption and Bone Density

It's probably not a big surprise that even bone density responds better to a well-rounded, healthy diet. Recent research from Tufts University, published in the *American Journal of Clinical Nutrition*, has revealed that taking calcium and vitamin D supplements and eating a well-balanced diet, as well as maintaining a *moderately* high protein intake, increases bone density. Participants taking placebos, instead of the calcium and vitamin D supplements, showed bone loss regardless of protein intake. A separate study at Tufts University found that men who eat a well-balanced diet high in fruits, vegetables, and cereals had higher bone density than those who had poorer diets.

77

## Supplements That May Aid Absorption

### Vitamin D

There may be many supplements that aid in the absorption of calcium, but vitamin D is considered to be the most necessary. The hormone calcitriol, also called "active vitamin D," cannot be formed without sufficient amounts of vitamin D. Insufficient calcitriol, in turn, causes insufficient calcium absorption from the foods we eat. When the body does not absorb enough calcium from the diet, it gladly takes what it needs from our bones. This weakens the skeleton in two ways because not only is the calcium being taken from the bones, but it also prevents the formation of any new bone.

There are two ways to get vitamin D: through the skin—from exposure to the sun—and from the foods we eat. Vitamin D is formed naturally in the body after exposure to the sun. If you live in a sunny place, such as Southern California, and spend even a moderate amount of time outdoors just by going from a store to your car, you probably don't need to worry about your vitamin D intake. It only takes 15 minutes of sun per day for your body to produce and store the vitamin D that you need. If you think you may not spend that much time outside everyday, or if where you live is eternally cloudy and you have very short winter days, then you will want to consider taking a supplement. The recommended daily intake of vitamin D is 400–800 International Units (IU). Vitamin D is not water soluble (your body will not get rid of excess through the urine), so don't overdo it. Massive doses of vitamin D can be harmful.

### Foods High in Vitamin D

| | | |
|---|---|---|
| Cheese | Butter | Margarine |
| Cream | Fortified Milk | Oily Fish |
| Oysters | Fortified Cereals | Eggs |

### Zinc

Zinc is a trace mineral that contributes to cell division and growth—important for creating denser bones where we are trying to encourage the osteoblasts to lay down new bone cells, to increase bone density.

### Foods High in Zinc

| | | |
|---|---|---|
| Beef | Pork | Lamb |
| Poultry | Peanuts | Peanut Butter |
| Legumes | | |

## Manganese

Manganese supplements support proper growth and health. While a manganese deficiency has never been found in humans, manganese deficient animals show improper bone and cartilage formation. A manganese deficiency may also contribute to growth problems.

### Foods High in Manganese

| | | |
|---|---|---|
| Whole Grains | Cereal Products | Lettuce |
| Dry Beans | Peas | |

## Vitamin K

Vitamin K has been getting a lot of positive press lately for its use in increasing bone density. Studies have shown that it aids in maintaining strong bones because of the protein—osteocalcin—that it produces. Osteocalcin aids in bone remodeling, thus becoming an aid in increasing or maintaining bone density. A study performed at Maastricht University in the Netherlands found that high doses of vitamin K greatly decreased bone loss in post-menopausal women. The Framingham Heart Study and the Nurses' Health Study have both established an association between high vitamin K intake and decreased hip fracture risk. Surprisingly, Americans' average intake of vitamin K is on the low end of the scale. Perhaps taking a supplement or eating foods high in vitamin K might be in order for you, too.

### Foods High in Vitamin K

| | | |
|---|---|---|
| Cabbage | Cauliflower | Spinach |
| Broccoli | Soybean Oil | Cereals |
| Soybeans | Canola Oil | Lentils |
| Green Leafy Vegetables | | |

Note: The gastrointestinal tract also produces vitamin K.

## Magnesium

More than half of the body's magnesium is found in the bones, where it is essential to bone metabolism. Magnesium also directly influences the function of bone cells. There have not been sufficient study's on magnesium to prove its worth in preventing bone loss or improving bone density, but it is, in general, considered a necessary nutrient for bone health.

### Foods High in Magnesium

| | | |
|---|---|---|
| Avocados | Spinach | Broccoli |
| Potatoes | Bananas | Kiwi Fruit |
| Chocolate | Nuts | Seeds |
| Peas | Beans | Cereal Grains |

### Potassium

Certain studies, such as the Framingham Heart Study, have found a positive effect on bone density when magnesium and potassium are used together. The combination of these two supplements prevents blood from acidifying. This effect is beneficial because higher acid levels in the blood result in more loss of bone cells through resorption as the calcium is leached away.

### Food High in Potassium

| | | |
|---|---|---|
| Artichokes | Spinach | Potatoes |
| Bananas | Squash | Tomatoes |
| Meat | Fish | Lobster |
| Milk | Yogurt | Lentils |
| Orange Juice | Broccoli | Cantaloupe |

## Easy Recipes for Higher Calcium Intake

Are you having trouble getting enough calcium in your diet through the foods you eat? Here are some family recipes I found in my kitchen that may help give you some ideas of how you can incorporate higher calcium meals and beverages into your everyday eating. Following the recipes, are simple ideas that you can slip into your diet for even more calcium intake. Most of the recipes are relatively fast and easy, so it won't take you a lot of time to give these new ideas a whirl.

### Appetizers and Salads

#### Fried Cheese

| | |
|---|---|
| 1/3 cup margarine | 1/2 lb. Jarlsberg cheese, shredded |
| 1 tsp. prepared mustard | 2 egg yolks |
| dash salt | 2 eggs |
| 1/4 tsp. pepper | 1 cup plain dried bread crumbs |
| 1 cup flour | vegetable oil |
| 2 cups nonfat milk | |

In a medium saucepan, over medium heat, add the mustard, salt, pepper, and 2/3 cup flour. Mix well. Add milk and cook until thick. Add cheese, stirring until smooth. In a separate bowl, beat two egg yolks. Add two tablespoons of the hot cheese mixture to the egg yolks. Stir, and then pour into cheese mixture. Refrigerate 4–8 hours.

In a shallow dish, beat the remaining two eggs. Place 1 cup each of flour and bread crumbs in separate shallow dishes. Take the refrigerated mixture and form small cheese patties that are about 1/2 inch thick. Dip the patties in the flour, then the egg. Finish in the bread crumbs. Refrigerate for about 1 more hour. Just before you are ready to serve the patties, fry them in oil over medium heat until lightly browned on both sides. Serve with spaghetti sauce, salsa, or guacamole.

### Mom's Salmon Ball

8 oz.   cream cheese (use Neufchatel for lower fat)
1 Tbs. onion, minced
2 Tbs. horseradish
dash   Tabasco sauce
2 cans salmon (5 oz. each) **or** 2 cans of shrimp (4.5 oz. each)

**For sauce:**

5 oz.   chili sauce                     juice   1/2 lemon
dash   Worcestershire sauce      1 tsp.   horseradish

Mix cream cheese, minced onion, 2 tablespoons of horseradish, and Tabasco with salmon or shrimp. Form a large ball and refrigerate.

Mix chili sauce, lemon juice, Worcestershire, and the remaining teaspoon of horseradish. Pour sauce over salmon ball. Refrigerate until ready to serve. Serve with crackers.

### Yogurt-Cheese Dip

8 oz.   Neufchatel (lowfat)        1/2 cup plain, nonfat yogurt
1/8 tsp. dill                            1/4 tsp. salt
Favorite vegetables for dipping

Mix the cheese, yogurt, salt, and dill until smooth and chill until you are ready to use.

### Broccoli Slaw

16 oz.  broccoli slaw mix           1 cup   sugar
1/2 cup apple cider vinegar       1/4 cup water
1/2 tsp. dried mustard              1/2 tsp. celery seeds

Place broccoli slaw in a large bowl. Combine the sugar, vinegar, water, mustard, and celery seeds in a small saucepan. Boil over high heat. Allow the mixture to continue to boil as you stir constantly. Remove from heat once the sugar has dissolved. Pour hot mixture over broccoli slaw. Refrigerate until well-chilled, stirring occasionally.

### Easy Greek Salad

2     medium cucumbers, peeled and sliced

6 oz.  (1 can) Greek olives, drained

2     green onions, chopped

1/2 lb. feta cheese with herbs and garlic, crumbled

1 tsp. Oregano leaves

salt and pepper to taste

2     large tomatoes, chopped into wedges

2 oz.  (1 can) anchovy fillets, drained (optional, but very high in calcium)

2 Tbs. capers

olive oil and balsamic vinegar

Combine all ingredients, mix well, and enjoy.

## Breakfast

### Swiss and Broccoli Quiche

1     pie pastry

4 oz.  shredded Swiss cheese

2 cups heavy cream

dash  salt

1/2 Tbs. butter

4     eggs

16 oz.  (1 bag) frozen broccoli florets

Beat together eggs, cream, and salt. Stir in cheese. Pour into prepared crust that has been placed in a 9-inch pie plate. Add broccoli florets. Bake for 15 minutes at 425 degrees. Turn oven down to 325 degrees and bake for an additional 35 minutes.

### Scrambled Eggs and Shrimp

4     eggs

4.5 oz. (1 can) shrimp, drained

1/8 cup milk

1/4 tsp. prepared mustard

Beat together the eggs, milk, and mustard. Add shrimp. Spray a skillet with nonstick cooking spray and cook egg mixture over medium heat. Serve with bagels or toast. Salt and pepper to taste.

## Main Dishes

### Salmon Pasta Salad

16 oz. (1 can) salmon, drained

16 oz. broccoli florets

2 cups edamame (soybeans)

Lowfat or fat free Italian dressing

12 oz. pasta of choice

1     each red and yellow bell pepper, chopped

Cook pasta, broccoli, and edamame as directed. Toss together all ingredients except salad dressing. Refrigerate for 2 hours. Add salad dressing to taste.

## Fish Tacos

| | | | | |
|---|---|---|---|---|
| 3/4 lb. | fresh salmon | | 1.25 oz. | (1 package) taco seasoning |
| 1/2 head | romaine lettuce, chopped | | 3 | large tomatoes, chopped |
| 8 oz. | (1 package) shredded Mexican style cheese | | 2.25 oz. | (1 can) sliced olives |
| | | | 12 | taco shells |
| salsa | | | sour cream | |

Sprinkle the taco seasoning on top of the salmon. Bake in a 9 x 13-inch baking dish at 350 degrees for 12 or 15 minutes or until light pink and flaky. (If you are running short on time, you can toss it in a resealable plastic bag with some olive oil and microwave it for 4 or 5 minutes. Be sure to leave a little opening in the bag for hot air to escape.) Put all of the remaining ingredients in separate bowls and call everyone to the table! To layer your taco, first put the salmon in the bottom of the shell, followed by the lettuce, tomato, cheese, olives, salsa, and sour cream.

## Easy Pizza

| | | | | |
|---|---|---|---|---|
| 1 | prepared pizza crust | | 14.5 oz. | (1 can) pizza sauce |
| 1/3 lb. | lean ground beef, browned and drained | | 2 oz. | (1 can) anchovies, drained (optional, but high in calcium) |
| 8 oz. | shredded part-skim mozzarella | | 1 | large tomato, very thinly sliced |

Spread the sauce over the pizza crust. Top with ground beef and anchovies. Sprinkle on the cheese and top with tomatoes. Bake at 450 degrees for 8-10 minutes.

## Sweet and Sour Shrimp

| | | | | |
|---|---|---|---|---|
| 1 1/2 lb. | cooked medium shrimp, deveined | | 1 cup | dried long grain rice |
| 1 | each red and yellow bell peppers, chopped | | 40 oz. | pineapple chunks (2 cans, 20 oz. each) |
| 1 clove | garlic, minced | | 1 Tbs. | cornstarch |
| | | | 1/2 tsp. | ginger |

Cook rice according to package directions. Pour pineapple chunks into large skillet, reserving 1/2 cup of pineapple juice. Add cornstarch to reserved juice and mix until all the lumps disappear. Add peppers and shrimp to the skillet, and bring to a boil. Add cornstarch/juice mixture to skillet. Simmer until thick. Serve over rice.

## Mary's Pierogies

**For filling:**

2 1/2 lb. farmer cheese              4 small potatoes, mashed

1/2 lb.   cheddar, shredded

Combine, cover and refrigerate overnight.

**For dough:**

8 oz. sour cream                     3 cups  flour

3     large eggs                     1/4 cup butter (1/2 stick), melted

Mix dough until smooth and elastic. Working with half of the dough at a time, roll on a floured surface until thin (ravioli thin). Cut squares approximately the width of your hand. Put two or three tablespoons of filling on each square. Fold the square to make a triangle and press to seal. As you are preparing them, cover them with a damp towel so they won't dry out. Place about 5-6 pierogies at a time in a large pot of boiling water. Boil until pierogies float. Remove to a platter and cool. The kids in my family prefer these with tomato sauce; the adults prefer fried onions and sour cream as a topping.

This recipe makes several dozen. What you are not ready to eat, freeze before boiling. When you are ready to eat them, just toss them in a pot of boiling water.

## Baked Macaroni and Cheese With Tofu

16 oz.  (1 package) elbow macaroni      18 oz.  (1 package) firm tofu

1 tsp.    salt                          3 Tbs.  butter

1         small onion, minced           2 Tbs.  flour

1/2 tsp. dry mustard                     1/4 tsp. pepper

3 cups  nonfat milk                      4 cups  shredded cheddar cheese

Preheat oven to 350 degrees. Cook macaroni according to package directions and drain. Toss crumbled tofu in with the pasta. In a medium saucepan, over medium heat, melt 3 tablespoons of butter. Add minced onion to saucepan and cook until soft. Add flour, mustard, pepper, and salt to onions. Stir until smooth. Add milk and stir until thickened. Remove from heat and add cheddar. Place macaroni and tofu in 9 x 13-inch baking dish. Cover pasta with cheese mixture. Bake 20 minutes.

## Beverages

### Hot Vanilla

*I like chocolate, but I love vanilla! Try this for a nice warm drink instead of hot chocolate.*

1 1/2 cups nonfat milk                     1/4 tsp. vanilla extract
1 1/2 Tbs. sugar

Pour all of the ingredients into your favorite microwave-safe mug and heat for 1 minute or until desired temperature. Stir until the sugar dissolves. Enjoy!

### Milkshakes

1 cup    nonfat milk                 1/2 cup  fresh fruit to complement
1 cup favorite ice cream                      your ice cream flavor (cherries
                                              with chocolate, bananas with
                                              strawberry, etc.)

Place all of the ingredients in a blender and blend until smooth.  Pour into a tall glass and you are all set.

### Root Beer Float

12 oz. (1 bottle) or can of your      1 scoop  vanilla ice cream
        favorite root beer

Put the ingredients together for a frosty treat that is high in calcium. You can use diet root beer and frozen yogurt for a treat that is lower in calories.

### Eggnog

3            eggs, separated          1/4 cup sugar
1 1/2 cups milk                       ground nutmeg
1/4 cup    heavy cream

In a large bowl, use a mixer to beat egg yolks and sugar. Continue to beat for 15 more minutes or until the mixture is thick and lemon-colored. Be sure to keep scraping the bowl to thoroughly mix.

Chill. Just before serving, combine yolk mixture, milk, and 1/3 teaspoon nutmeg. In a separate bowl, use the mixer to beat egg whites until soft peaks form. In a small bowl, using the mixer again, beat heavy cream until stiff peaks form. Gently fold egg whites and cream into yolk mixture. Fold until just blended. Serve with a sprinkle of nutmeg on top.

This recipe makes about 5 servings.

Desserts

### Regina's Banana Split Bars

**For crust:**

| | |
|---|---|
| 3/4 cup margarine, softened | 3 cups graham cracker crumbs |

**For topping:**

| | |
|---|---|
| 1 cup margarine, softened | 2 cups powdered sugar |
| 1 tsp. vanilla extract | 2 cups heavy cream |
| 6 or 7 bananas | 2 eggs |
| 1 large can crushed pineapple in juice | sliced almonds (high in calcium) maraschino cherries |

Mix together 3/4 cup margarine and the graham cracker crumbs. Press evenly on a cookie sheet. Bake at 350 degrees until browned (10–15 minutes). Cool completely.

Using a mixer at medium speed, beat together remaining 1 cup of margarine, sugar, and vanilla for 20 minutes. Spread on crust. Slice bananas lengthwise (three slices per banana). Dip bananas in lemon juice and place on sugar mixture. Drain pineapple and place over bananas. Beat the heavy cream at high speed until you have whipped cream. Spread the whipped cream over the bananas and pineapple. Top with almonds. Use the cherries when you are ready to serve.

## More Ideas for High Calcium Eating

Try these ideas for sneaking more calcium into your diet:

- Pineapple chunks with cottage cheese for lunch.
- Oatmeal with milk instead of water.
- Homemade bread made with milk instead of water.
- Orange juice fortified with calcium.
- Broccoli with a sour cream dip.
- Cook and serve edamame (the soybeans you can find in the frozen food section of your grocery store) in the pod. It's fun to shoot them in your mouth—my son loves them that way. Or serve them already shelled, as a side dish to any dinner entrée.
- Bagels with Lox and Cream Cheese. (Lox is cured, smoked salmon, very popular in New York. You can find lox at most of the popular bagel chain stores nationwide or in most grocery stores. When my mother serves lox, she also serves fresh tomatoes, lettuce, onions, and capers to go along with it. Very, very yummy. If you've never heard of lox, don't feel bad. I grew up in a very small town and had friends who had never even heard of bagels.)

- Tofu in your spaghetti sauce, lasagna, or eggplant parmigiana—because tofu is bland, it takes on the flavor of whatever you put it in. You can sneak it in to almost anything for a calcium boost.

- Powdered milk in your soup and casseroles.

- Almonds, sesame seeds, or sunflower seeds strewn on all of your salads.

- Sardines on your bagels, or in sandwiches—try them! You actually may like them, and they are a great calcium source.

- Nonfat plain yogurt with your favorite fruit—lots of calcium and you'll avoid the sugary content of those yogurts that already have the fruit added

- Pretzels wrapped in your favorite cheese.

| Sample Menus for Higher Calcium Intake | | |
|---|---|---|
| **Menu 1** | **Menu 2** | **Menu 3** |
| **Breakfast** Oatmeal with milk. Orange juice with calcium. | Bagel with lox and cream cheese. Orange juice with calcium. | Scrambled eggs and shrimp. Orange juice with calcium. |
| **Lunch** Cottage cheese with pineapple chunks. 8 oz. milk. | Grilled cheese sandwich. 8 oz. of milk. | Eggplant and tofu from a local Chinese restaurant. |
| **Dinner** Fish tacos with salmon. | Easy pizza with anchovies. | Salmon pasta salad with broccoli. |
| **Snacks** Hot vanilla or hot chocolate made with milk. | Frozen yogurt. | Pretzels wrapped in your favorite sliced cheese. |

## Happy Eating and Talk to Your Doctor

There you have it. These ideas for adding calcium and other important supplements to your diet should get you started on the path to improved bone health. You should, of course, talk to your doctor before making any changes in your diet. Especially ask your doctor about adding supplements to your diet, because it is always possible that supplements will interact adversely with your system or a medication that you may be taking. Remember, natural does not always mean safe.

# Chapter 5

## All That Stuff Your Doctor Said: Medication for Building Bone Density Made Easy

"Screening for osteoporosis through a directed history and bone mineral density scanning should be a part of every perimenopausal woman's comprehensive medical evaluation. Commitment to an appropriate exercise program and adequate calcium supplementation are the cornerstones of osteoporosis prevention.

For women with significant osteopoenia or frank osteoporosis, additional treatment is available. As the pendulum again swings away from the routine use of hormonal replacement therapy as a means of osteoporosis prevention and treatment, alternative medications are moving to the forefront. Foremost among these are the biphosphonates, namely Alendronate ([brand name] Fosamax) and Risendronate ([brand name] Actonel)."

—Kathleen Bundy-Anderson, MD, of Santa Clarita, California

We're rolling now! Onto the third part of your four-part plan for fighting osteoporosis—medication. Many of you are probably already taking a medication for osteoporosis that was recommended by your doctor. Great! Read on to find out exactly why it helps. For those of you considering medication, the information that follows will give you an idea of what is available. You can then talk to your doctor about what is best for you.

There are several medications that are approved by the U.S. Food and Drug Administration (FDA) for treating bone loss. Some are better suited for a person who has suffered bone loss due to hormonal changes and aging. Others are better suited for bone loss due to certain medications that have caused the bone loss. To begin with, why don't we look at what is available for treating osteoporosis. The diagrams that follow describe the different classes of drugs that treat osteoporosis and what they are meant to accomplish. A very important note here is that this information is in *absolutely no way* meant to take the place of your doctor's advice. In other words, don't demand medication from your doctor. Discuss it with him or her to come up with the best solution for you. I compiled this information only to save you research time, seeking data on the types of medications available. This is not advice or even a suggestion as to what you should be taking in the way of medication for treating osteoporosis. Talk to your doctor!

# Common Medications for Treating Osteoporosis

The following four charts give a very brief overview of the four most common classes of medications that are currently being used for treatment of osteoporosis.

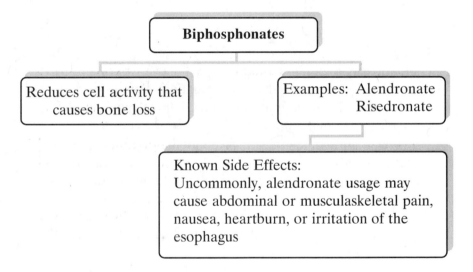

## More on Biphosphonates

Alendronate (brand name "Fosamax") and Risedronate (brand name "Actonel") have both been shown to slow or stop bone loss, increase bone density at the hip and spine, and reduce fracture risk overall. Alendronate was originally approved for treating secondary osteoporosis caused by glucocorticoid treatments, which are used for treating inflammatory ailments like rheumatoid arthritis (to see a list of illnesses treated by glucocorticoids see page 26).

Alendronate has recently been approved for all forms of osteoporosis and has received very high ratings. In a six-month study comparing Alendronate to Risendronate, the former was more effective in halting bone loss. With Alendronate, a 150 percent greater increase in hipbone mineral density was found, as well as a 50 percent greater increase in lumbar spine bone mineral density than with Risendronate. Another study found spinal fracture risk to be reduced by almost 50 percent with Alendronate. Alendronate has also proven to be faster, more effective, and to have a lower drop out rate than Risendronate because it can be taken once a week rather than every day.

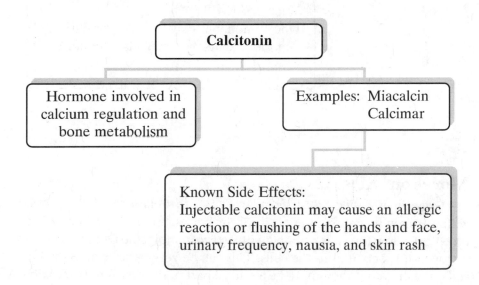

## More on Calcitonin

This non-sex hormone has been shown to slow bone loss and increase bone density in the spine. Some anecdotal information claims that calcitonin has also relieved the pain due to fractures in many patients. Both spinal and hip fractures may be reduced with calcitonin. The results are not back on the fracture risk studies as of yet. Besides the injectable form of calcitonin, there is also a nasal spray. A runny nose has been the only reported side effect of this calcitonin spray. Studies have shown that calcitonin is less effective than estrogen replacement therapy or Alendronate in slowing bone loss, increasing bone density, and reducing fracture risk. It is also more expensive than estrogen.

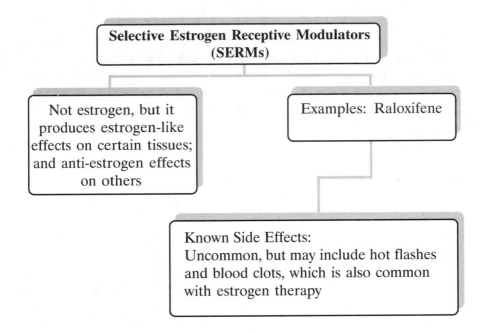

## More on SERMs

Sometimes called "designer estrogens," this class of drugs interacts with estrogen receptors in the cells of the bones, breasts, and heart. These receptors allow the cells to bond with estrogen molecules, thus turning on estrogen-like activities in the cells. This can be very beneficial in the bone cells, as estrogen is thought to be a crucial part of the continual breakdown and rebuilding of bone cells. Studies are now underway to find ways to make SERMs react with only certain estrogen receptors—such as in the bones, to increase bone density—but not with breast and heart estrogen receptors, where estrogen is linked with breast cancer and heart disease.

Tamoxifen, a SERM approved two decades ago, was used as a treatment for breast cancer. Unfortunately, it was found that while this drug combated breast cancer, it increased the risk of endometrial cancer and serious blood clots. On the other hand, Raloxifene does not increase the risk of endometrial cancer and is being investigated as a means of breast cancer prevention.

### Black Cohosh as a SERM

Black cohosh is a popular phytoestrogen (sometimes called a "plant estrogen") used for treating menopausal symptoms. Researchers have found that it may also be a SERM. Besides showing benefits in treating menopausal symptoms, such as hot flashes and vaginal dryness, researchers noted that black cohosh seemed to activate the *osteoblasts*—cells in the bone that create new bone. Although black cohosh is presently an over-the-counter supplement, do not assume that it is the remedy for you. Phytoestrogens have been shown to have the same effects on body tissues as estrogen. This could mean that you are raising your risk of breast cancer by taking a phytoestrogen. Talk to your doctor—even about over-the-counter, "natural" supplements.

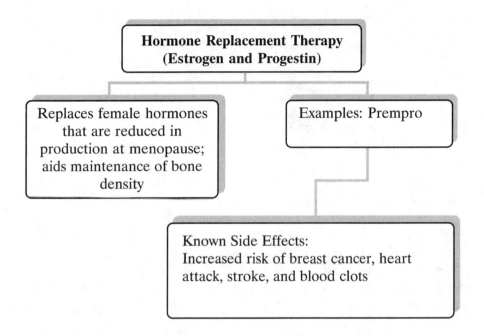

## More on Hormone Replacement Therapy (HRT)

The Women's Health Initiative (WHI)—a study of 16,608 women taking either estrogen and progestin or a placebo over a period of five years—reported in July of 2002 that the risks of hormone replacement therapy far outweighed the benefits for many women (the benefits being decreased risk of hip fracture and colorectal cancer). The study was initiated to investigate the benefits of estrogen on the heart and in the reduction of hip fractures in menopausal women. It had been widely believed that estrogen reduced the risk of heart disease. However, scientists found that estrogen is actually harmful to the heart. Because of the increased risks, not only of heart attack, but of breast cancer, stroke, and blood clots, scientists abruptly halted the study (three years short of its original completion date in 2005). Combined estrogen/progestin therapy taken by women with a uterus showed these risks and benefits:

- 41 percent increase in strokes.

- 29 percent increase in heart attacks.

- 100 percent increase in blood clots in legs and lungs.

- 37 percent less colorectal cancer.

- 34 percent fewer hip fractures.

- 24 percent less total fractures.

A current study by the WHI will now assess the risks and benefits of estrogen-only therapy. These results will be available in 2005.

### Increased Risk Still Small

Scientists working on the Women's Health Initiative, while agreeing that the study was properly and prudently halted due to increased risk factors, were also quick to note that the increases were small. For example, out of 10,000 women, there were only eight more cases of stroke (which is a 41 percent increase over what was found in the placebo group), seven more cases of heart attack, 18 more cases of blood clots, and eight more cases of breast cancer. Still, this is a notable increase, especially if you are one of the 8 more people who get breast cancer. However, some women, if they are considered to be at low risk for these diseases, may opt to speak to their doctors about maintaining a hormone regimen.

### Hormone Replacement Therapy: Always Refused by the Majority of Women

Until now, HRT was strongly recommended for treating hot flashes, building bone density, maintaining skin elasticity, and other menopausal concerns. But it was never very popular with women. After the results of the Women's Health Initiative were published, even more women began to research alternative treatments, such as exercise, for their menopausal symptoms. Even before the study's findings were published, only a third of premenopausal and menopausal women chose HRT. The other two-thirds had reservations about the benefits of HRT and feared an increased risk of breast cancer. These women decided, even then, that the side effects of HRT were too adverse. They also felt that treating menopause with drugs was too much like treating a disease. Menopause is a normal transition in a woman's life, and they felt it could be treated with more "natural" alternatives. For more on this subject, see Chapter 2.

### Your Own Estrogen After Menopause; A Little Extra Fat Can Be a Good Thing!

After menopause, although levels of one form of estrogen—estradiol—drop, one form of estrogen—estrone—continues to be produced. The site of estrone production is largely in fat tissue, aided by the adrenal glands. Although this form of estrogen is weaker than the estradiol produced by your ovaries, it increases with age and with the amount of fatty tissue. That little bit of extra fat that you may have put on once reaching menopause is helping your body to produce its own estrogen. The weight gain may be an example of your body naturally doing what's best for you. Of course, be careful not to add too much fat. You don't want the risks to outweigh the benefits!

### Low-Dose Estrogen and Its Benefits

Scientists have found that a low dose of estrogen (.25 milligrams of estradiol, as opposed to the regular dosage of 1.0 milligrams) decreased bone loss in a study performed on women 65 years old and over. One study, published in 2000 by the *Journal of Clinical Endocrinology and Metabolism*, by lead author Karen Prestwood, M.D., stated that there was an increase in bone density without the normal side effects of a higher dose of estrogen therapy, which include breast tenderness, headaches, bloating, and fluid retention. But what about the increased risk of cancer from taking estrogen? A study, published in *Lancet* in 2002, showed that low-dose estrogen taken vaginally caused no increase in endometrial cancer. However, if taken orally, the risk of endometrial cancer increased by 300 percent, and abnormal endometrial cell growth was increased by 800 percent.

## Additional Options

Outside of the four medical treatments outlined above, additional options have recently been developed. These alternatives are currently under investigation for their potential effectiveness in reducing bone loss and rebuilding bone density.

## Natural Estrogen and Progesterone

It is not known if the natural estrogens on the market today are any safer than the chemically compounded estrogen/progestin combination that was studied in the Women's Health Initiative. However, it is known that these natural estrogens are chemically identical to the hormones that a woman's body produces.

Popular chemically compounded hormone replacement therapy drugs take their estrogen from the urine of pregnant horses. My sister was more than a little amused when she called me a few years ago to tell me her doctor wanted to give her horse urine for her perimenopause symptoms!

Instead of the chemically compounded estrogen, natural estrogen and progesterone are available. Natural estrogen and progesterone are derived from plants like wild yams and soy. All three forms of estrogen that a woman's body produces—estradiol, estrone, and estriol—are obtainable in formulas known as *TriEst* (a triple natural estrogen) and in *BiEst* (a dual natural estrogen). Natural progesterone can also be found in similar formulas. Drug companies are jumping on the bandwagon and also making natural estrogen products now. Their products, such as Estrace (a pill) and Estraderm (an estrogen patch) contain only estradiol—not estrone and estriol.

Some anecdotal reports describe natural estrogens as being more effective than traditional hormone replacement therapy because of their chemical arrangement. Some view that alternative methods of administering natural estrogens, such as the skin patch and micronizing techniques, may make the natural estrogens more effective. The skin patch bypasses the liver and enters the bloodstream directly, possibly making it safer. Micronized progesterone, made from finely ground yams, is thought to be much more easily absorbed and therefore more effective. Micronized progesterone is currently available under the brand name Prometrium.

Doctors have warned, however, that there is no current basis for belief that these natural estrogens are any less dangerous than the traditional hormone replacement therapy. It could be that all forms of estrogen that are added to a woman's system are going to have the same positive *and* the same negative consequences.

## Androgen Therapy

Androgens, a class of hormones that include testosterone, are generally thought of as male hormones, the same way estrogen is considered a female hormone. Contrary to this belief, women's bodies actually produce a considerable amount of androgens. Unlike estrogen, androgens do not decline abruptly at menopause. Instead, they begin to decline in a woman's late 20s and slowly diminish until they are at about 50 percent of their peak levels by menopause. A woman who has had an oophorectomy, where the ovaries are surgically removed, can have her androgen levels drop rapidly to less than 80 percent of peak levels.

When androgens decline at their normal, gradual rate, the effects of their loss are not as readily apparent as the uncomfortable symptoms associated with rapidly declining estrogen levels that occur at menopause. Because androgens are associated with dense bones, more muscle mass, and a healthy libido (among other things), scientists feel that an androgen supplement could very well be the answer to some menopausal symptoms—including bone loss. Studies are currently underway to find out if an estrogen/androgen therapy would be helpful to postmenopausal women.

Recently, testosterone has been offered to women who do not get relief from hot flashes and vaginal dryness through estrogen replacement therapy. Just as estrogen is often combined with progestin, a newer hormone replacement therapy combines estrogen with testosterone (brand name "EstraTest").

Androgens can also be found in supplements such as DHEA. Because supplements are not regulated by the FDA, some of the supplements have high androgen levels, while others have negligible levels of the hormone. Remember, natural does not mean safe. Do not treat yourself with DHEA before talking to your doctor.

One of the concerns about treating women with androgens is their masculinizing side effects. These can include a lowered voice and facial hair (which sound like more than a *concern* to me—although I guess neither is life threatening). On top of that, all androgens have the potential side effect of liver injury, fluid retention, acne, sleep apnea, aggressive behavior, and the lowering of HDH (good) cholesterol. Androgens pose a potentially very beneficial path for hormone replacement therapy in the future. For now, though, there is still much research to be completed.

## Biochemical Markers

Scientists can use biochemical markers to find out specific information about how your bones are developing—or not developing, as the case may be. The markers provide specific information about bone resorption back into the bloodstream and bone formation for denser, stronger bones. A doctor could potentially use these markers of bone turnover to understand how rapidly you are losing bone. Perhaps you are what the medical world defines as a "rapid loser." Most women lose bone mass at a rate of 1 percent each year during menopause, but "rapid losers" lose 3–5 percent every year. If there was evidence that you were rapidly losing bone density, you could begin taking an osteoporosis medication for prevention before developing dangerously low levels of bone density. In other words, you would be targeted as high-risk for osteoporosis and preventive measures could be taken.

Biochemical markers could also be useful once you have begun a treatment plan. Doctors can determine in just months if the medication you are on is working. If you saw positive clinical results in just 12 weeks or so, wouldn't you feel better about taking the medication? You would know it was working. Doctors would also know if the therapy was not working, or if you stopped taking the medication (no more fibbing about how loyally you took your meds).

Even though this technology exists, biochemical markers of bone turnover are not in widespread use. You can find them in use at the offices of many specialists in bone density for determining bone loss and effectiveness of therapy, but they do have limitations. For example, they are not a substitute for measuring bone mineral density. You may see them more in the future, but for now, scientists are still working on making them useful for the evaluation of individual patients.

## Sodium Fluoride

Most osteoporosis medications increase bone density by decreasing bone loss. These types of medications enable the bone tissues to retain calcium, making it is less likely to be reabsorbed into the bloodstream. Sodium fluoride, on the other hand, may increase bone formation. Sodium fluoride as a possible treatment for osteoporosis is not a new idea. In fact, a study performed more than 40 years ago found a correlation between osteoporosis and small amounts of sodium fluoride in drinking water. Although, it is not yet approved by the FDA, it shows promise as a future treatment.

Scientists Watts and Blevins, of the Emory School of Medicine in Atlanta, Georgia, studied the effects of 25 milligrams of slow-release sodium fluoride taken with a calcium supplement, on 100 women with osteoporosis. The study results showed that the women increased their bone density by about 5 percent over 14 months. The control group taking the placebo did not show any improvement. Also, new vertebral fractures were almost nonexistent in women taking sodium fluoride. Because the side effects appear to be much lower for slow-release fluoride than they are for other fluoride treatments (sometimes resulting in stomach and intestinal difficulties), it seems that slow-release sodium fluoride could potentially be a future treatment for osteoporosis. Unfortunately, the same study showed that for women with very low bone density, bone mass did not increase with sodium fluoride treatment. There was also no apparent prevention of the continued deformity of vertebrae that have already fractured in these same women with very low bone density. It seems that, once the disease progresses to a certain state, it does not respond as easily to efforts to stop its progression. Talk to your doctor to see if this treatment has been approved by the FDA yet, and to see if you may be a good candidate.

# A Note From Your Dentist:
# Teeth Are Bones, Too

There is little research in the area of how osteoporosis affects the bone density of the jaw and teeth, but there seems to be a correlation. Osteoporosis doesn't just affect the spine, hips and wrists. Those are the most common sites for fracture, and they are, therefore, given the most attention. But all of the bones, including the teeth, are affected by reduced bone density. In one study, conducted in 1996 by Krall, Garcia, Dawson-Hughes, and associates, scientists found that as normal bone loss occurs as we age, so does the risk of tooth loss. It seems that the bone that holds our teeth in place (the alveolar process) becomes diminished with osteoporosis, and therefore, the teeth can become loose and fall out.

Because scientists assume that a correlation exists between osteoporosis and tooth loss, they believe that dental x-rays may be a good source of information when looking for osteoporosis in a patient. In 1996, scientists from the University of Washington School of Dentistry found just that. Their x-rays were very accurate in determining which patients had osteoporosis and which had normal bone density.

## Estrogen and Your Teeth

Because estrogen increases spinal, hip, and wrist density, it almost goes without saying that it will also increase the density of the bone in your jaw. Bone loss in the jaw, besides loosening the hold on your teeth, is going to make you more susceptible to *periodontitis*—an infection of the gums that is a common cause of tooth loss. As the space around the teeth increases, so does the possibility of infection. In the Framingham Heart Study, scientists found that those women taking estrogen had many more teeth than women not taking estrogen. As I stated earlier, not many studies have been done on bone density and tooth loss. It may be that some of the other medications available for osteoporosis could have the same results of preventing tooth loss as estrogen. Talk to your doctor.

# In Closing, on Medications

There is new information available all the time about the possibilities for improving bone density with medication. Stay up to date about what is most effective and safe by talking to your doctor and by keeping your eyes and ears open for new information available through the media. Also, keep your doctor informed of any medical changes or other risk factors (see Chapter 1 ) that may put your bone density in jeopardy.

# Part Two

## OsteoPilates Exercises

# Chapter 6

## Go! Go! Go!: A Little Motivation to Get You Started

This chapter is where I get to be your personal cheerleader! There is a reason that personal trainers, like aerobic instructors, are stereotyped as being jolly little souls with enough energy for themselves and 20 other people. So if you need a little encouragement, a bit of a jump-start, or you are having trouble staying motivated, this section is where you can turn. As I said in Chapter 1, you are already a motivated, take-control, self-reliant person, or you would never have bought this book in the first place. This already puts you in the category of the type of client I love to see. You have already taken the first step—you have chosen to manage and direct your health. No one has the power to change the quality of your life but you. However, there are cheerleaders out there, such as personal trainers, to get you going in the right direction.

This chapter will review why exercise increases bone density, what "the OsteoPilates 7" mean to you, and how to get started and stay motivated.

## The Piezoelectric Effect—Not a Disco Move

Resistance training has been proven effective in building bone density and treating osteoporosis—they call it the piezoelectric effect. Any time your muscles are stressed (as with exercise), they, in turn, put stress on the bones. This stress stimulates the bones to grow, becoming denser and thicker—a good kind of stress. If you were to never exercise, your bones would become thinner and more prone to fracture.

Resistance training has been shown to not only increase bone density, but also to halt bone loss due to resorption. OsteoPilates is resistance training. The resistance you will be using is gravity—your own body weight. In some instances, light hand weights can be added to augment certain exercises. So if someone asks you what the heck you're doing when you start your new exercise program, you can tell them, "I am doing the piezoelectric effect!" Words with five syllables will catch anyone's attention.

# The OsteoPilates 7

The OsteoPilates exercises found in Chapter 8 for people with normal bone density, and the exercises in Chapter 7 for people with low bone density (osteopoenia and osteoporosis), address seven factors that are of special concern to the exerciser who is trying to increase bone density. Also referred to as the "OsteoPilates 7," these factors include:

1. Increased bone density.

2. Powerful "core" strength.

3. Improved balance.

4. Enhanced overall strength.

5. Better flexibility.

6. Improved posture.

7. Perfect alignment.

## #1—Increased Bone Density

For patients with osteoporosis, doctors often recommend starting an exercise program because of the piezoelectric effect of exercise. A 1997 study by Kohrt, Ehsani, and Birge further revealed that bone density can be increased by resistive exercise such as OsteoPilates. In addition, the study found that the increase in lean body mass and strength, gained from specific exercise forms like Pilates, was important in preventing osteoporotic fracture by reducing the risk for falls.

## #2—Powerful "Core" Strength

Every Pilates exercise is designed to involve the body's abdominal and back muscles together, also called the "core." In essence, every Pilates exercise is an "abdominal exercise." So if you are working the arms, in particular, you are also working the core. When you work the legs, you work the core. In fact, you don't even need to do one sit-up to have a strong core. This focus on the core makes Pilates the perfect exercise for someone with osteoporosis, because it is these central muscles that support the alignment of the spine, which increases balance and reduces falls.

## #3—Improved Balance

The older we get, the more we become concerned with our ability to balance. We begin to realize that it may not be as easy as it used to be to balance. Falling becomes a lot scarier with the increased risk of serious injury that aging brings. For osteoporotic patients, balance is of an even greater concern because a fall can result more readily in a fracture. Balance is increased with OsteoPilates because of its focus on abdominal ,or "core," strength, and because the exercises gradually develop and increase balance. Like many things in our lives, our balance improves with practice.

Improved abdominal strength as a result of OsteoPilates improves those muscles at the center of your body that "catch" you or pull you back to an upright position when you feel yourself slipping or starting to fall. Your proprioception, or your perception of where you are in space, will also improve with practice. This will prevent falls from happening in the first place.

## #4—Enhanced Overall Strength

The 100-year-old exercise form that is Pilates, has become extremely popular in the last few years as the general population has caught on to this best kept secret of professional dancers. Dancers have used Pilates for more than 60 years to create strong muscles that are flexible and not bulky. As you work toward your bone-building goals, you will also be building a stronger, longer, leaner physique. In OsteoPilates, all of the exercises involve more than one part of the body at a time. This allows for overall strengthening and toning, with a relatively small number of exercises. Your new strength will give you more energy and greater ease of movement in everything you do (this means less aches and pains).

With clients who have suffered any sort of injury, there is a pattern that I see frequently (to which I fell victim myself, when I injured my back). When people are injured they don't want to exercise—not a big surprise when someone is in pain. Unfortunately, extended lack of exercise results in additional muscles becoming weakened, resulting in more aches and pains. When I hurt my back, I stopped exercising for a period of a couple months. When I finally started again, not only was my back hurting, but my shoulders, neck, and knees were giving me trouble. I felt like I was coming apart at the seams—everything hurt. That pain was a result of my entire body having become weak. I see similar patterns over and over again with my clients. So if something hurts, don't necessarily stop doing *everything*. Avoid what hurts, and keep doing what you can. Your body will thank you. A happy body will, in turn, keep your mind a little happier and peppier.

## #5—Better Flexibility

Many of our poor posture habits are due to inflexible muscles. Tight shoulder muscles pull the upper back forward into a "hunched" position—an osteoporosis "no-no" (see Chapter 3). Tight thigh muscles, or hip flexors, can pull the low back out of alignment, making it more difficult to maintain proper alignment in the upper back. Maintaining these misalignments, over time, can result in pain. Improving flexibility can relieve pain relatively quickly when the pain is caused by inflexible muscles. Added flexibility has made a big difference for many of my clients. Many notice an increase in the ease of movement and/or reduction of pain in their daily activities, within the first couple weeks of starting their program.

## #6—Improved Posture

A primary focus in Pilates is improving posture. Posture refers to how you routinely position and hold your spine throughout your daily activities. "Postural awareness" comes about by doing these exercises with proper posture. Good posture should apply not only when you are standing, but also when you are kneeling, sitting, or lying down.

It is necessary to take the time to make sure you are performing each detail of every exercise correctly, even if it means doing fewer exercises per workout, initially. Quality, *not* quantity, counts. Guidelines for correct posture are included with each exercise. You can also refer to the "Reminder Glossary" at the end of the book. This glossary elaborates on the "Reminder Photos" included with each exercise. It will help you better understand how to perform each exercise with the proper posture.

## #7—Perfect Alignment

Alignment refers to the physical placement of all the body's parts in relationship to each other. Ideally aligned, your body is balanced, centered, and using the minimum amount of energy necessary to stack one body part on top of another. Good posture is a big part of proper alignment, but it's not everything. Placement of the legs, shoulders, and arms also come into play when evaluating alignment. When I am evaluating a client's execution of an exercise, I even consider the placement of the feet on the floor or the position of the feet when the legs are pointing toward the ceiling. Sometimes, to a new client, it seems nitpicky and even annoying. However, it is this exact attention to detail that makes Pilates as effective as it is. In your OsteoPilates program, it is not good enough to do it "sort of right." Read and follow all of the instructions that go with each exercise, and you'll get the maximum results.

# Getting Started and Staying Motivated

Below, you will find an assortment of tips, bits of information, challenges, and some good old advice to help you get going. Before the advice, though, let's start with what you'll need to begin a Pilates mat program.

## You, a Little Space, and a Mat

Getting started on your OsteoPilates program is pretty darn simple, not to mention exciting. All you'll need is yourself (dressed comfortably), a mat (or not), and the floor. I prefer using a mat (you can find one at your local sporting goods store) to prevent my hip and shoulder bones from grinding into the floor as I exercise. Also, a designated OsteoPilates mat makes what I am doing a little more special. If my family sees me pull the mat out and then lie down (and this is the important part), they know to leave me alone for awhile. Even the dog seems to know not to come rolling around on me when I have the mat out, for fear of an errant toe in her face. You may eventually want to get some small hand weights to enhance certain exercises and make them more challenging. Don't overdo it, though. One- or two-pound weights can make an exercise significantly harder.

## The Second Most Frequently Asked Question

People first ask me what kind of equipment they'll need to start an OsteoPilates program at home (we just covered that). Secondly, they want to know how often they'll need to do their exercise program in order for it to be effective—to experience results. The answer is: Perform your exercise program three times a week to experience change. Exercising up to five times a week is fine. Exercising more than that will put you at risk of over-exercising and either burning out your interest, or burning out your body. Body burnout often shows up in the form of tendonitis, pulled muscles, body aches, or fatigue. The joints and muscles have been overworked and have not been given time to heal.

Once-a-week exercising, occasionally, is okay for maintaining what you have built, but will not add anything (strength or bone density) to what you already have. Keep this in mind, in case you are ill one week, too busy, or traveling. You can maintain what you have and can then start adding to that when your schedule returns to normal.

## "No Pain, No Gain"—the Fallacy

Yes, a challenge is necessary, but don't overdo it. The fitness motto, "no pain, no gain," is quickly dying out and it is about darn time. Exercise physiologists have given this old motto the boot because studies have proven that pain after exercise is unhealthy.

In Pilates, there has never been a motto of "no pain, no gain." And if you think you have to suffer in order to look good, just walk into any Pilates studio and look at the instructors. They look great (long and lean, not bulky), and they haven't been killing themselves like an overachieving, under-trained gym-rats. The most important thing to remember is: "Great amounts of pain result in great amounts of dropouts" (not to mention injury). People who are in pain as a result of an exercise program don't generally go back to it until the muscle soreness is gone. Those people might never return to such an unpleasant experience. Even if you could get them to go back, the layoff and/or damage they endured would have them starting over again from square one. And that, my friend, is the real reason for avoiding pain. If you don't want to derail your exercise program, don't kill yourself to the point that you can't exercise at all.

## Exercise Feels Good

What? You don't think so? You could be doing it wrong. When I lived in snowbound Park City, Utah, I used to love to go cross-country skiing. Whenever I told people where I was off to, I would invariably be accosted with groans of, "How can you do that? It's too much work!" or "I tried that once and it was miserably difficult." I always told them that they were just doing it wrong. To cross-country ski correctly, you have to grab a few friends, some grapes, cheese, and crackers and head out to the middle of nowhere. You shuffle along on those skis while looking around at some of the most gorgeous scenery on Earth. When you are tired, stop and eat. Then shuffle some more, laugh with your friends, eat some more, and ski some more. How could you possibly have a bad time?

Exercise in your everyday life should be the same way—enjoyable. Grab a few friends and some snacks (why not?) and have a party. If you are executing a well-balanced exercise program, as well as performing the right amount of exercise for your fitness level and experience, then exercise *does* feel good. While you exercise, your shoulders release, your chest opens up, and you feel lighter, more awake, and taller. However, don't ruin these moments of well-being by overdoing it. If you don't look forward to exercising, you probably are working too hard, or your program is imbalanced. Start out slowly and build up. I know that patience can be hard when you are excited about starting something new, but trust me—"slow but sure" definitely wins the exercise race.

## Are You Over 25?

I hate to be the one to tell people this, but here goes: Did you know that at age 25 we begin to lose muscle mass at the rate of a half pound of muscle per year? Did you also know that because of this reduction in muscle mass, your metabolism begins to drop by about 4–6 percent every 10 years or so? Yikes and double yikes! Fortunately, you will always have the ability to increase muscle mass throughout your life. So if you haven't exercised in awhile, your rate of improvement will be off the charts! That's the good news. You'll see results quickly and start feeling better almost immediately. Your energy level will be greatly improved and the aches and pains due to years of inactivity will subside. On the other hand, if you continue to not exercise, you will gradually become weaker, less toned, and less able to perform everyday activities without needless pain and stress on your body.

## Stick to It

Why do so many people begin an exercise program with complete dedication, only to become a statistic in the dropout ranks? Dropout rates are usually due to asking too much of yourself all at once. Many people who begin a workout program in my studio want everything *now*. They want their abs to hurt, they want slimmer thighs, and they are discouraged when they do not see physical changes by the end of the second week. Joseph Pilates has a famous quote that begins, "In 10 sessions, you'll feel the difference…" The 10 sessions he was speaking of are usually over 5 or 10 weeks. Many of my clients report feeling the difference almost *immediately*, so 10 sessions is a pretty safe bet. In Pilates, you are retraining yourself into a new lifestyle and movement philosophy. Your body doesn't just become stronger as you perform the exercises—it becomes healthier and more balanced. Give yourself some time.

## How to Get Down to the Floor

I know it may sound odd, but the hardest part of starting a mat program can be getting all the way down to the floor. No, I don't mean in the physical sense—that the knees may creak and the hips may ache, not to mention the back. I mean in the sense of just lying down in order to get going, start exercising, and move those bones! Sometimes when it's time for my clients to do their home program, they tell me that they just can't make themselves get started. I tell them they need to lie to themselves (just a little white lie) and say that they are going to lie down and do just one exercise, such as the breathing exercise on page 123. It'll feel good to relax and relieve a little stress. Now, once you are down there and relaxed, I guarantee that you'll feel like doing more than just breathing. Tell yourself, "two more exercises," and then "two more," and then "two more." If you end up doing only two exercises on a night when you are especially tired, that's okay. That's two more than you would have done, otherwise.

## Don't Keep It Simple

Your bones need a physical challenge in order to increase density. If you do the same exercises over and over, what may have initially been a challenge to you and your bones, will become easy. That's good—you've gotten stronger. The body is an amazing thing, and your bones, like your muscles, answer to the challenge and adjust to whatever you give them to do. In fact, our bodies are incredibly responsive. They will try their best to do whatever we ask.

So after awhile, throw some variety and a challenge or two into your routine, to go beyond maintenance and to further increase your strength and bone density. Spice it up! If you've been doing the beginning OsteoPilates program, move up to the intermediate as soon as you're ready. If there are just one or two exercises that are too easy, then add one or two pound hand weights to those exercises. Having said all that, remember: You don't have to be in pain to be challenged or to increase bone density.

# So, You've Hit a Plateau

Is there an exercise that you'd really like to be able to do, and you just can't seem to get it to look like it does in the book? Some clients struggle with flexibility of the *hamstrings*—the muscles at the back of the legs. Others struggle with upper back mobility or range of motion at the shoulder joint. Whatever it is for you, we all have body parts that just don't want to go where we'd like to put them. So what do you do? Do you just accept that you'll never be able to do that particular exercise? This is the part where I am supposed to say, "Of course you can do it! Nothing will stop you!" Well, maybe, and maybe not. Read on!

## Getting That Exercise Perfect

Let's begin with those of you who have no physical limitations inherent in the makeup of your body. In other words, you know that you do not have anything that might prevent you from trying to do a certain exercise. If you know there is nothing preventing you physically from your goal then, yes, we can get over this plateau. No need to worry. For example, let's take an exercise that combines flexibility and strength—Double Leg Stretch (page 135), for those with osteoporosis or normal bone density. Let's say you can't get your legs as straight (pointing toward the ceiling) as you'd like or as low as you'd like. What can you do? First you need to find what muscle group is preventing you from getting where you want to go. It seems fairly obvious that the lack of flexibility in the hamstrings may be preventing you from being able to straighten the legs. However, it could be the weakness of the *hip flexors*—the muscles that are at the crease in your hip—or lack of abdominal strength that is preventing you from achieving your goal. As a further example, lowering your legs to the floor takes more than just abdominal strength. You are going to need back strength and flexibility to brace your spine as the legs lower. Taking these examples into consideration, you could add exercises to your routine that focus on hip flexor strength (such as Side Kicks IV, page 159), stomach strength (such as Toe Touches, page 173), and back strength/flexibility (such as Swan I, page 167).

## When You Shouldn't Push Too Hard to Achieve a Goal

Sometimes, whether or not you will be able to do a certain exercise depends on what your body has given you to work with. For instance, where the upper back should be slightly curved, mine is very flat. As a result, during many shoulder exercises, my shoulder blades protrude off my back in a somewhat abnormal way, sometimes called "wings." I was initially told it was because I had a certain muscle group that was weak. Finally, a qualified physical therapist told me it's not. I just have a flat back and will always have "wings." Not a big deal, unless someone tries to "fix it." So, if you have one shorter leg, scoliosis, severe *kyphosis* (a rounded or humped upper back), a fused spine, or any of a number of other slight variations of the human body, don't beat yourself up over not accomplishing every task. Just accept what you can do and keep going.

You do, however, want to be sure that your self-diagnosis is correct. Some people, as many chiropractors will tell you, think they have one leg longer than the other, when actually they have a muscular imbalance in the spine, which is hiking one hip up higher than the other, making one leg appear longer. One thing you can do is keep working on the problem areas. Even though my back is flat, I do give it a little push in a rounder direction. On each inhale, I try to push it into the mat. Conversely, for a rounded upper back, keep doing your spine extension exercises, such as Swan I, Swan II, Double Leg Kicks, Single Leg Kick, and Swimming (pages 167, 169, 133, 161, and 171). All of these exercises will help you to reduce the curve in your upper back and provide muscular balance. For scoliosis, keep working on the Mermaid (page 145) and the Saw (only for those who have normal bone density—page 204). You may never be able to bend as far on one side as the other, but keep working at it. Just as with a curved upper back, the more you balance the muscles, the less pain and discomfort you will experience.

## Stamina

If stamina is an issue for you—if you can't get through an entire exercise program or get to a new level—then consider these factors:

1. Don't push yourself too hard, too fast.

2. Do the entire program, broken up into smaller pieces throughout the day.

3. Make those pieces of the program bigger and bigger each week.

4. Move through the program more slowly, resting for 30 seconds to a full minute between exercises.

You may also want to add walking to your exercise regimen. I am a big believer in the health benefits of walking. Walking improves your aerobic capacity. If your aerobic capacity increases, then your stamina for your strength program will also.

# How to Keep the Exercise Fire Burning

Even if you have exercised your entire life and religiously follow your OsteoPilates program three times a week, you'll have days or even weeks where you just don't want to exercise. Some will exercise anyway, but others will just stop completely until the motivation returns. So how can you keep your motivation working for you all the time?

Most of the time, when people feel their interest waning, it is a result of boredom due to a lack of challenge, change, or goal. There are several ways to combat waning interest. Grab a friend and have her exercise with you. Knowing that your friend is waiting for you to show up at her house to exercise may give you that extra push out the door. Even people who will let themselves down by not exercising won't let a friend down who is waiting for them.

Of my clientele that has been coming to my studio for more than a year, 70 percent are in a group class. They know their classmates are going to exercise whether or not they show up. Motivation from one's classmates can be powerful, as most of my clients love each other's company. Also, no one wants to fall behind. (They don't want their friend's stomach to look flatter than their own!)

However, the ultimate motivations my clients cite, are the aches and pains they experience performing routine activities after a 2- or 3-week Pilates layoff. Move it or lose it.

Another method of self-motivation is setting goals. Do you have a party on the horizon that you'd like to look good for? How about someone in your life that would appreciate and congratulate you on your new, improved body? That someone doesn't have to be a husband or wife. Hopefully, we all have friends that would be happy to see us looking and feeling better.

## Just Think Dessert

If all else fails to return your interest in exercise, just think dessert. Think chocolate cake, oatmeal cookies, homemade bread, or gourmet meals that are usually 50 percent butter. Exercise boosts your metabolism (remember the previously mentioned decline in metabolism). A higher metabolism raises the amount of calories your body burns, even when you are reading, watching television, or just sleeping. If you exercise, at least when you do indulge, you won't feel guilty.

Many of my clients say that they are hungry after exercising, but don't want to go home and eat, canceling the good work they've done. This logic is wrong on several levels. First of all, your body is going to burn the most calories after exercise, in the first half-hour, while it is still warm and revving from your workout. Secondly, you don't want to put your body into starvation mode. If your body is unsure of when you are going to feed it (such as if you have very irregular eating hours), it will start hoarding what you do feed it. Your body's priority is survival. It doesn't know that you are going to feed it in another 5 or 6 hours. It is worried about *now*.

So if you go long stretches without eating, chances are very good that your body won't let go of a single calorie without a fight. In other words, your irregular eating habits are forcing your body into a slower metabolism. If you want to boost your metabolism, eat regularly—small meals throughout the day. The purpose of an exercise program is to feel better and to be healthier. How can your health possibly improve if you don't eat reasonably when you are hungry? Of course, the opposite is also true. How can your health possibly improve if you eat junk when you are *not* hungry?

## Making Time to Exercise

Lots of people call me to inquire about Pilates, only to tell me at the end of the conversation that they, "just don't have time to exercise right now." They say they'll get back to me after the New Year, summer vacation, or Groundhog Day. I know what it's like to be busy. I know what it's like to have every minute of the day scheduled so that running through my day (clients, family, life) is like operating a finely tuned instrument. My sister says that my name, "Karena," means "she who doesn't return phone calls." And I admit that there are weeks where one more phone call, one more trip to the market, or one more client seems impossible. Still, I have made exercise a priority. It's a choice, just like happiness. You can be an optimist or a pessimist. You can also be a physically fit and healthy person, or not. The choice is truly yours.

The nice thing about exercise is that the payoffs are predictable. If you exercise three days a week, you are assured certain results. Physical improvement is not based on anyone else's permission, approval, or opinion. It's all about you and what you want your body to do. I don't believe that people are basically lazy. I think people give in too easily to television, a cup of tea, or an excuse. However, there is not a single person who has walked through my door who has not said that it feels good to move, to stretch, and to awaken once-dormant muscles. That's not laziness. That's recognizing an innate need to be strong, healthy, and vital.

# Figuring Out Why You Exercise

Knowing why you exercise can be a huge help in increasing your chances of continuing to exercise. Obviously, you are wise enough to be concerned about your bone density. That, all by itself, keeps many of my clients going. They refuse to give in to a disease that has been proven to respond positively to exercise, medication, and diet. They refuse to give in to what many health specialists call "the most easily preventable disease." But there are more reasons to exercise than just bone density. What are those reasons for you? I encourage you to think about this one when you are out on a walk, writing in a journal, or meditating.

I know why I exercise, and it may have nothing to do with why most of my clients exercise, mostly because I don't do it for a flatter stomach or thinner thighs. I used to, but I gave up—I was never satisfied with those goals. My stomach was never flat enough and my thighs never thin enough. So to continue to keep my spirit for exercising, I had to dig a little deeper. You should too. It will keep you exercising for the rest of your life and you'll improve the quality of your life. I could tell you why I exercise, but then you might be tempted to take those reasons as your own. Besides, you already know why you exercise. Just think about it for a minute.

# Your Health, Your Life

If you have ever had an injury, or if you are currently recovering from an osteoporosis fracture, then you know how difficult it is to separate who you really are from the pain your body is feeling. Psychologists tell us that we are not our bodies. We have the power to separate how our bodies feel from how we perceive ourselves. I know when I was recovering from two herniated disks, I tried to do just that. My back may have been causing me chronic pain, but I was pushing forward, despite the throbbing discomfort. I refused to allow myself to become, "that lady with the bad back."

Your health is your life. No matter how valiant a battle you wage to put pain aside, sometimes the pain remains and continues to affect your day-to-day living. However, pain can be reduced, and I believe that fitness plays a big role in that. I'm speaking of overall fitness that can change the way you feel, as opposed to a few stomach exercises and a few bicep curls.

If it is a part of your body, then it needs to be moving. I have several clients with bad knees, who have only done leg lifts to improve the strength of their knees. Leg lifts only work one part of the *quadriceps* (thigh muscles). Once I get them working on all the parts of the quadricep, as well as *all* of the muscles of the leg (back, sides, and front), they begin to have more strength and less pain in their knees almost immediately. I also get them working on every other muscle that can be exercised, from the neck to the shoulders, hands, stomach, back, and feet.

Once given an overall exercise program, my knee clients experience less pain in their knees, specifically, and in their entire bodies, in general. They are able to walk farther, thus live better and, in turn, feel better. Whether I have a client with bad knees or just the general "glitches" that come with age, the exercise programs I provide keep them less stiff, more flexible, more vital, and more alive. Sometimes, managing pain is a matter of raising your quality of life. Being able to enjoy a day is a great motivation to exercise.

# An Experiment of One

You are your own experiment. What will this program do for you? Will your bone density increase? Will you feel better? Will you look better? Will you have more energy? Will you be more excited about life? Will you look forward to outings that you had formerly dreaded? Will you relish your newfound strength and be anxious to use it and to challenge it? I have had clients answer yes to all of these questions. Whether you will too is yet to be seen. But it's time to get going and see what you can do for you. My thoughts for a healthier body are with you. You can do it—good luck!

# Talk to Your Doctor

You should, of course, talk to your doctor before beginning any exercise program. Review this book with your doctor and be sure that he or she feels it is appropriate for you at this time. She may have additional directions or restrictions. You and your doctor should be partners as you work your way to better health. Be sure to keep him informed about what you are doing.

# Preliminary to Starting Your Exercises

I have a few hints for getting the groundwork correct before beginning your exercises. The following tips will make every exercise work more effectively to help you reach your goal more quickly. Attention to detail is a significant factor in why Pilates is as effective as it is. Don't skip these details!

## Global Conditioning: What's Good for the Abs Is Good for the Calves

Men and women alike tell me, "I want to get rid of this roll," as they grab a slab from around their stomachs. "More stomach exercises!" is the cry I hear. I have two things to say to these stomach people (and if you are one of them, *please* listen!):

1. Strong muscles can be firm muscles, but can only flatten so much. If your stomach is protruding too far over your jeans, then you also need to lose fat.

2. Working one part of your body exclusively imbalances the rest of your body. Imbalance causes pain. For instance, in a well-rounded Pilates program, an abdominal exercise is shortly followed by a back exercise. Not only is this opposite muscle group strengthened to balance the strength of the abdominals, but the abdominals are stretched at the same time.

## Get to the "Core" Now!

The core is such an important part of every Pilates exercise that, before starting your Pilates program, you need to find your core. Once you know the location of your core, you'll know what muscles should be involved in each and every exercise.

### Just Cough

The easiest way to find your core muscles is to place your hands just inside your hipbone and then cough. Did you feel the muscles that tightened? Those are your deep abdominal muscles. Those are the muscles that maintain your balance, support your lower back and organs, and—yes— flatten your stomach.

### Kissed Ribs and Bellybuttons Up and Under

The "Kissed Ribs" is a method I use with my clients to help them begin working the core muscles immediately. This exercise is important, not only for all of the following exercises, but for *all* of your everyday activities. I encourage my clients to practice Kissed Ribs throughout the day, everyday, to improve their alignment and posture and to begin shaping their abdominals. Kissed Ribs will do more for the overall shaping of your abdominals than all the crunches in the world. It's all about incorporating a low, consistent level of exercise into all facets of your everyday life.

### How It's Done

Let's start easy. First let's try Kissed Ribs lying down. Start with your knees bent, and soles of the feet down so that your heels are about 12 inches from your hips. Your hands should reach past your hips on the floor. Use the muscles just below your breastbone to push your spine flat into the floor. Even though the hips will be tipped toward you, do not use the hip muscles at all on this exercise. Your buttock muscles should feel very loose. With your uppermost abdominals pulling down, imagine that your ribs, on either side of those abdominals, are trying to kiss. This "kissed" feeling will keep your core working and your spine flat.

Now, without changing the position of the ribs or spine, carry both arms overhead. Most people are not flexible enough to allow the hands to touch the floor overhead if the spine is truly prevented from changing position. You should feel a tension between the lowest ribs where the stomach muscles are working and you may feel a stretch in the shoulders, particularly in the armpit area, if you do not allow the spine to change. The tension you feel is the abdominal muscles working to keep the ribs from splaying.

Many people, when they are told to stand up straight, immediately push the chest forward. Instead, the chest needs to stay in alignment. A forward thrust in the chest is going to result in the low back and legs compensating for the misalignment—which results in low back, hip, and even knee pain. In order to prevent this misalignment, you can imagine that the ribs just below your breastplate have been sewn together or are "kissed" together so that they cannot splay apart.

**Don't Splay the Ribs**

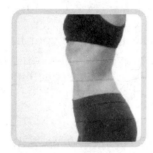

**Kiss**

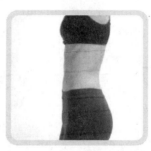

**Relaxed Abdominals**

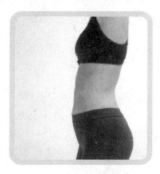

**Bellybutton Up and Under**

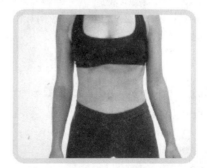

When correcting your posture, think more of lengthening the spine and drawing the top of your head to the ceiling instead of thrusting the chest forward. (It may make your chest look bigger, but your butt and thighs will also look much bigger as those muscles will be overworked in order to maintain some semblance of alignment to prevent you from falling on your nose.) You want a natural arch in the low back. Also, while standing, pull your bellybutton gently towards your spine and up and under your ribs. You should feel like your stomach muscles are lifting up and away from your hipbones. Once you get the hang of pulling the abdominals up and then under your ribs, you will visibly be able to see your bellybutton lifting or moving upward. The gentle pressure created on the abdominal muscles by closing the ribs in front (or by performing Kissed Ribs) will quickly help you to increase your core strength.

## A Little Extra Help for the Stomach

Did you see the section in Chapter 3 entitled "Abdominal exercise alert! Do them wrong and your stomach gets bigger!"? If you missed it, first go back and check it out. Then you'll be ready for the following information. The following guidelines can help you confirm whether or not you are doing an abdominal exercise correctly. The number one rule in abdominal work is: Never let the stomach pooch out. If you want to develop flat abdominal muscles (and who doesn't?), keep your stomach flat when you are exercising. Read on for tricks for flatness!

### You Are a Drum

Okay, not you, but your abdominals. Try this exercise while lying down. Imagine that your stomach muscles have been stretched across your hipbones. They are taut. They are flat. They do not bulge forward from the hipbones. Now, as you perform any of your exercises, try to keep your abs in this same, flat, tightened position. Keep your abs taut—do not relax them at all throughout the complete range of motion of the particular exercise. However, don't let your abdominals "bulge" forward as you flex them. This should not be a straining effort, but a gentle tension to hold the muscles taut and flat.

### Belly Dancer Roll
### (This is for people with normal bone density only!)

It can be extremely difficult to keep the stomach flat when you are rolling up and down in an abdominal exercise. Try this exercise, and you'll go beyond flat and look absolutely concave, while doing abdominal crunches.

Start by sitting up straight with the knees bent and soles of the feet down, with the heels about 12 inches from the hips. Now, don't begin rolling down yet, but pull the lowest abdominals—the ones 4 inches below your bellybutton—toward your spine. As you begin to very slowly roll down, keep the lowest abdominals pulled in. Now, pull in the abdominals that are 2 inches below your bellybutton. Keep them there, and add the abdominals just behind your bellybutton. Continue to roll down and keep adding an abdominal group 2 inches at a time. Roll down as far as you can go without allowing the lowest group of abdominal muscles to release. As you roll up, reinforce the abdominals starting just below the breastplate. Now reinforce the abdominals 2 inches at a time as you roll up.

Working this way is going to make your abdominal work much more difficult. You are probably not going to be able to do nearly as many if you are working correctly like this. You'll be spending less time on abdominal work but you'll be getting better results. You can't beat that!

### Protruding Stomachs and Poor Posture

Some people, whose stomachs hang over their belts, don't need to lose weight. They simply need to stand up straight. I see women, all of the time, who stand like they are wearing 5-inch heels. Their hips stick out behind them, their chests protrude forward, and their stomachs hang loosely forward from their ribs. Stomach muscles are designed to pull in and support the organs and brace the spine. Poor posture is not only making these women look fatter than they really are, but the lack of support for the spine typically results in back pain. If you feel you are at a good weight for your body type/height, and still think you have too much stomach, try the postural alignment exercise in Chapter 3 on page 67.

# Ready, Set, Go!

Okay, you know the 5 Golden Rules for avoiding fracture and how to stand up straight, work your core muscles, and keep your motivation going. Now it's time to exercise. Good luck and enjoy!

# Chapter 7

## OsteoPilates:
### *Exercise Programs to Increase Bone Density, Reduce Fracture Risk, and Look and Feel Great!*

## Balance

*Safe for low bone density*

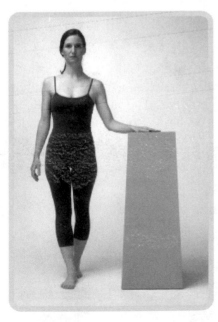 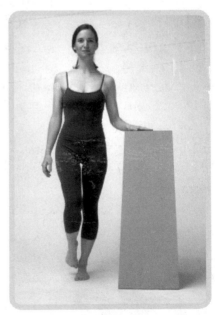

### Getting Started

Using a wall or countertop for support, stand with your feet together. Do not allow the toes to turn out or to face sideways.

## Moving

A. Step forward with one leg and place the heel of that foot against the toes of the other foot. Be sure to keep the toes of both feet facing straight ahead.

B. Slowly lift one leg off the floor. Only lift the leg as high as you can while maintaining good posture.

## Breathing

A. Take two slow breaths while holding the position and then put the other foot in front.

B. Inhale, lift the leg. Exhale, lower the leg.

## Repetitions:   8.

## Keep This in Mind

Do not allow the spine to slump forward or the hips to drop back as you are lifting the leg off the floor in version B. Usually, when the spine slumps it means you are bringing the leg up too high. Don't bring the leg up as high and keep the spine straight. This will make the core muscles work harder. Keep the shoulders wide and the core lifted.

## Picture This

Imagine that you are walking a tightrope. Be sure to use your arms for balance.

## Why Are We Doing *Balance?*

This exercise improves your sense of balance and coordination, which will reduce your risk of fracture. The balance muscles, just like any muscle group, get stronger and more adept with practice. The more you practice this exercise the better your balance will become. Your balance muscles are also your core muscles. A strong core reduces your risk of falling and lends a sense of ease to all of your movements of daily living.

## Reminders

For details, see the Reminder Glossary.

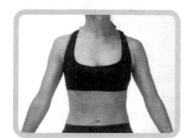
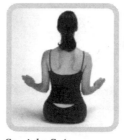
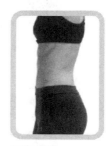

*Wide Shoulders*          *Straight Spine*          *Lifted Core*

**You don't want to look like this!**

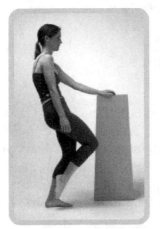

*If you are slumping while performing Balance, version B, you are probably lifting the leg too high. Lower the leg in order to keep the spine straight and the shoulders open.*

# Breathing

*Safe for low bone density*

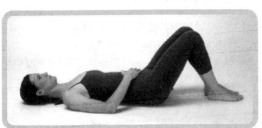

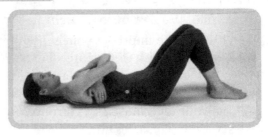

### Getting Started

A. Lie on your back, knees lifted, soles of the feet on the floor about hip-width apart and place one hand on your stomach just below your navel.

B. Same as version A except cross your arms over your chest so that you can feel your ribs with both hands.

### Moving

A. Breathe into your stomach so that the stomach fills up with air and expands on each breath. You should feel your hand being pushed up from the rise in your stomach on the inhale. You should also feel the low back pushing into the floor.

B. Breathe into the sides and back of your ribs. On each exhale, imagine that you are squeezing the lowest part of your ribs together to completely expel the air from your lungs.

**Repetitions:** 5 of each type of breathing.

### Keep This in Mind

If you are breathing properly, your chest and shoulders should not lift. If they do lift, you have an irregular breathing pattern called "accessory breathing." It is most common with smokers, individuals with chronic obstructive pulmonary disorder, back pain patients, and people whose stomach muscles are too tight to allow for the expansion on the inhale. Very tight shoulder muscles also contribute to the lift in chest and shoulders on the inhale.

Why should you change your breathing pattern? Studies have proven that breathing into the stomach or the ribs reduces low back, shoulder and neck pain.

### Important

With abdominal type exercises (all OsteoPilates exercises) you will want to use the B version of breathing. During the rest of the day, version A should be your natural way of breathing. If it's not, keep practicing version A and very soon you will be breathing into the stomach without even thinking about it.

### Why Are We Doing *Breathing?*

All muscles can become tight and inflexible over the years; this includes the diaphragm, which is our major breathing muscle. Proper breathing patterns need to be practiced. You may find that, the first time you practice breathing in these very particular ways, your stomach shakes or that your ribs feel tight. Your stomach and ribs may not move in the direction that you want them to at first. Keep practicing. Soon you'll find yourself breathing into your stomach and ribs naturally and without effort.

### Reminders

For details, see the Reminder Glossary.

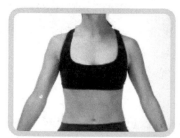 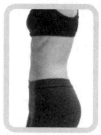

*Wide Shoulders*                 *Lifted Core (version B only)*

**You don't want to look like this!**

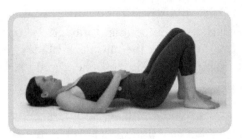

*Do not allow your shoulders to crawl up into your ears, and do not allow your back to arch away from the floor. Do not allow the chest to lift on the inhale.*

# Bridging

*Safe for low bone density*

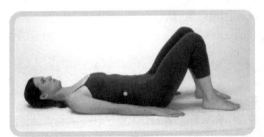

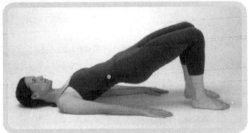

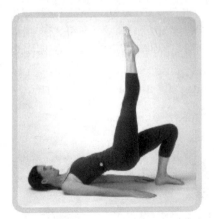

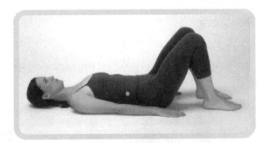

## Getting Started

Lie on your back with the knees up and soles of the feet down at hip-width apart. Lengthen the spine by imagining the tailbone and the crown of the head pulling away from each other in opposite directions.

125

## Moving

Keeping the spine as long as possible without curling the tailbone toward the ceiling, lift the hips up toward the ceiling. Only go as high as you are comfortable and don't go so high that the shoulder blades come off the floor. Now lower the hips back down. The tailbone should hit the mat at the same time as the low back.

## Challenge

When you can get the hips off the floor comfortably, try lifting one leg an inch off the floor, put it back down and repeat with the other leg. As you get stronger, lift the leg higher and begin to straighten it toward the ceiling.

## Breathing

Exhale, lift the hips. Inhale, lower back down.

## Repetitions: 4–8.

## Keep This in Mind

Rise up and down in one flat piece instead of vertebra by vertebra. Keep the shoulders on the floor and do not rise up onto the neck. Keep the inner thighs working by not allowing the knees to drop open.

## Picture This

Imagine that your entire trunk, from the hips up to the bottom of the shoulder blades, is a piece of wide, flat lumber. Stay flat and straight.

## Why Are We Doing *Bridging?*

This exercise extends the spine. Extending the spine will add strength and flexibility to the spine, which promotes better posture. As you will also be able to feel, this exercise strengthens the inner thighs and hamstrings, or the backs of the thighs.

## Reminders

For details, see the Reminder Glossary.

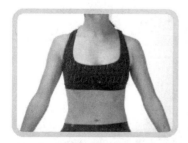
*Wide Shoulders*

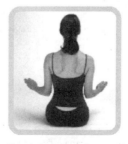
*Straight Spine*

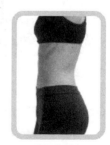
*Lifted Core*

**You don't want to look like this!**

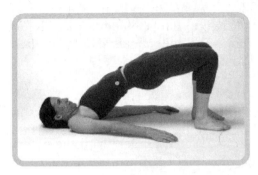

*Don't lift too high. Shoulders stay on the mat. Keep your shoulders pushing down your back; don't allow them to creep up into your ears. Don't allow the knees to drop open.*

# Chest Lifts

*Safe for low bone density*

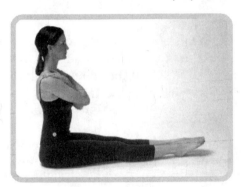

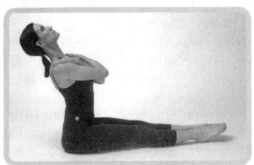

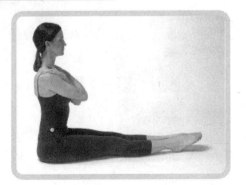

## Getting Started

Sitting with your legs extended straight out in front of you, or while seated in a chair, cross your hands to opposite shoulders. Sit with proper posture and with length in the spine. The abdominals should be lifted up and under the ribs without the shoulders lifting.

## Moving

Lift the chest toward the ceiling by arching the upper back. Be sure to isolate the upper back and do not change the shape of the neck or the low back.

## Breathing

Inhale, lift the chest. Exhale, return to your start position.

## Repetitions: 5–8.

## Keep This in Mind

It is very easy to allow the neck to do too much work on this exercise. Do not drop the neck back. It hurts and it's hard to breathe. The head and neck should only move back as a result of the chest lifting. If the shoulders lift or feel tight on this exercise, you are probably letting the neck drop back.

## Picture This

The place where your spine meets your neck should look like a gently curving C, not an L. The neck and head should look like a long extension of the spine, not a sharp turn in the road.

## Why Are We Doing *Chest Lifts*?

This exercise gives you more strength and flexibility for correct posture and reduced risk of fracture. Lifting the chest to the ceiling encourages flexibility in the upper back and across the front of the shoulders, while strengthening the muscles in the upper back and core. More easily attained correct posture will enable you to perform everyday activities with ease without flexing the spine (an osteoporosis no-no). Studies have proven that stronger spines are also less likely to fracture, even if the bone density is reduced.

## Reminders

For details, see the Reminder Glossary.

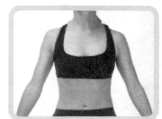
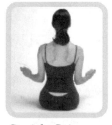
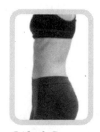

*Wide Shoulders*          *Straight Spine*          *Lifted Core*

**You don't want to look like this!**

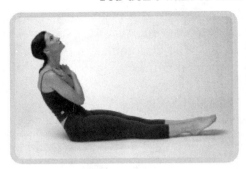

*Do not lift and jut the chin to the ceiling. Do not flex the spine. If you cannot straighten the spine with your legs extended in front of you, then perform this exercise while seated in a chair.*

# Puppet

*Safe for low bone density*

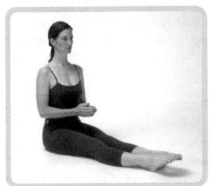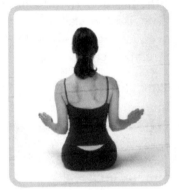

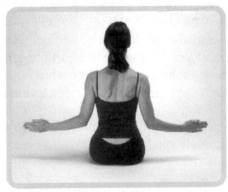

## Getting Started

Sitting with the legs extended in front of you, or in a chair, bend the elbows so they are at the waist and the forearms are parallel to the floor with palms touching.

## Moving

Open your forearms out to the sides of your body while gently squeezing the shoulder blades together. Return to the start position.

## Challenge

Add hand weights if you'd like. However, I find that this exercise is very isometric and I can increase the difficulty by squeezing the shoulder blades together a little harder.

## Breathing

Exhale, open the arms. Inhale, return to start.

## Repetitions:   12–16.

## Keep This in Mind

While performing *Puppet*, be sure to keep the spine in perfect alignment. Ideally, if you were sitting against a wall, you would feel your hips, shoulders, and the back of your head against the wall. Even though the elbows will not be able to remain touching the waist, the *intention* is to keep them there. If you cannot keep your spine straight while sitting on the floor, do this exercise sitting in a chair. This exercise is a great one to do if you have been sitting at the computer too long. You won't even have to leave your chair!

## Picture This

Imagine that your shoulders are tied to a chair but that your lower arms are free. Swing your arms in the available range or motion.

## Why Are We Doing *Puppet*?

The main emphasis of this exercise is to strengthen the muscles between the shoulder blades and to stretch the muscles at the front of the shoulders. This added strength and flexibility will improve your posture. Your risk of fracture will also be decreased because you will be better able to avoid a flexed spine. And don't forget that a stronger spine reduces your fracture risk. As with all of the OsteoPilates exercises, you are also working on core strength, which strengthens your stomach and spine.

## Reminders

For details, see the Reminder Glossary.

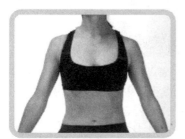 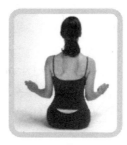 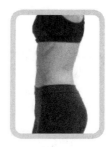

*Wide Shoulders*              *Straight Spine*              *Lifted Core*

**You don't want to look like this!**

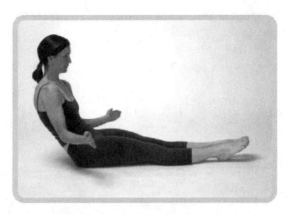

*Don't slouch. Keep your spine and the core lifted. Remember: Slouching puts you into a position of flexing the spine—a major no-no for osteoporosis!*

# Diamonds

*Safe for low bone density*

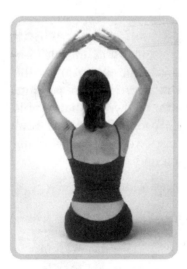
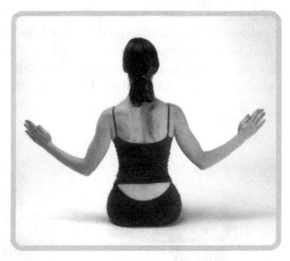

### Getting Started

Sit up straight in a chair, or with the legs extended directly in front of you. Your fingers should touch overhead with the elbows opened wide to the sides of your body. Gently pinch the shoulder blades together throughout the entire exercise.

131

### Moving

Lower the elbows to the waist. Return to the start position.

### Challenge

Add hand weights for an extra challenge for your shoulders.

### Breathing

Inhale, lower the elbows. Exhale, pause. Inhale, return to start. Exhale, pause.

**Repetitions:**   8–10.

### Keep This in Mind

Be sure to do this exercise in a chair if you can't straighten your spine with your legs straight out in front of you. Either way, keep the core lifted in order to keep strengthening those muscles, which will help you to maintain perfect posture. The shoulder blades should feel like they are always slightly pinched together. Avoid rounding forward at the shoulders.

### Picture This

Diamonds are a girl's best friend. In this case they keep you from having a stooped posture.

### Why Are We Doing *Diamonds?*

This exercise improves posture and reduces fracture risk. The muscles in the upper back and the abdominals are being strengthened in order to reduce a rounded or slumped posture. Keeping the shoulder blades pinched together will encourage flexibility at the front of the shoulders. This is very important since most of us have very tight shoulders due to driving, computer work, cooking, and cleaning—all of which pull our shoulders forward.

### Reminders

For details, see the Reminder Glossary.

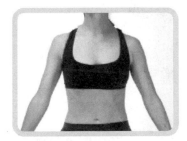
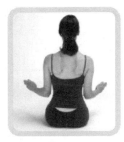
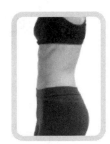

*Wide Shoulders*                 *Straight Spine*                 *Lifted Core*

**You don't want to look like this!**

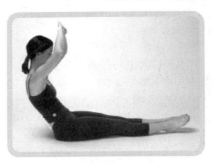

*Don't slouch. If your spine is slumped, as in the photo, you are flexing the spine (an osteoporosis no-no). Do not jut the chin forward. Your chin should be parallel to the floor and pulled gently in.*

# Double Leg Kick

*Safe for low bone density*

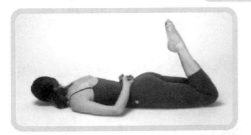

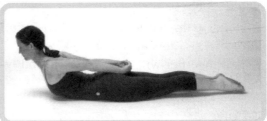

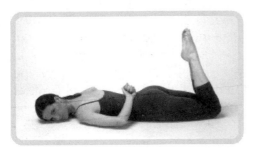

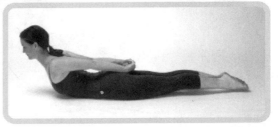

### Getting Started

Lie on your stomach and look to your left. Clasp your hands behind your low back and drop your elbows toward the floor.

### Moving

Bend your knees so that the heels come toward the hips. Double kick or pump the heels next to the hips. Now lengthen the legs back toward the floor as the arms reach long toward the feet. As the arms reach long, the head, shoulders, and chest come off the floor. Finally, lower the upper body and come back to your start position, looking to the right this time.

### Breathing

Exhale, double pump the legs. Inhale, lift the chest off the floor.

### Repetitions: 5–8.

### Keep This in Mind

The head and neck should be an extension of the spine. If you are not lifting the chest very far off the floor, you should not be looking up or in front of you as you lift. Even if you are able to lift the spine very high, you probably should only be looking at the floor about 2 or 3 feet in front of you, not straight ahead. Remember, do not put a crook in your neck by looking up too high with your eyes.

### Picture This

Imagine that your hands are holding on to a rope that is attached to a winch that raises your upper back as your arms pull toward your feet.

### Why Are We Doing *Double Leg Kick?*

This exercise is to strengthen and stretch the spine as well as strengthen the backs of the legs, or hamstrings. When you lift your back off the floor and extend your hands out toward the hips, you are encouraging proper posture. Better posture, as well as spine strength, lowers your fracture risk.

### Reminders

For details, see the Reminder Glossary

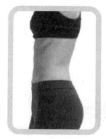

*Lifted Core*

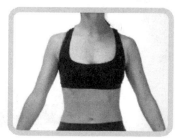

*Wide Shoulders*

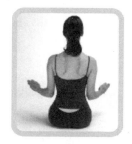

*Straight Spine*

**You don't want to look like this!**

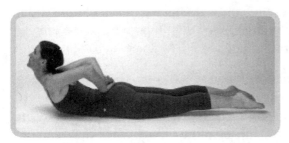

*Don't look up too high. Keep the head in line with the spine. Straighten the legs completely when you lift the chest. Keep the knees together when the legs are bent, as well as when they are straight.*

# Double Leg Stretch

*Safe for low bone density*

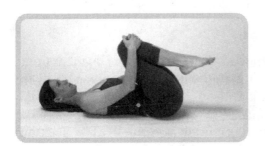

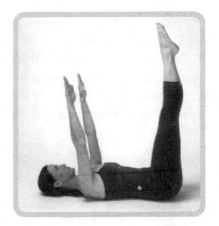

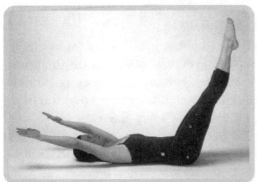

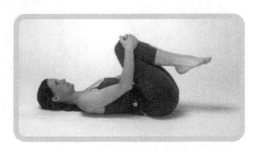

### Getting Started

Lie on your back with your hands and feet pointing directly to the ceiling. It is important that your knees be directly over your hips to begin the exercise, even if you have to bend the knees a little. Keep the spine flat on the floor.

### Moving

Move the arms and legs away from each other as you lower both toward the floor. Next, swing the arms wide to the outside of your body and down to your hips (like making an angel in the snow). Once the hands are down by the hips, bring the arms and legs back to their start position.

### Breathing

Exhale, open the limbs away from each other. Inhale, return to start.

### Repetitions:  4–8.

### Keep This in Mind

Do not let the spine release from the floor. Only lower the legs as far as you can while keeping the spine in contact with the floor. Even if you are quite strong, the legs won't go very low if you are truly working to keep the spine from moving away from the mat. Also, imagine that the crown of the head and the tailbone are being stretched away from each other. That image will keep your spine long and not crunched.

### Picture This

Imagine that your favorite cat or little child has come to sit on your stomach. Now your stomach can't lift and your spine can't release from the floor.

### Why Are We Doing *Double Leg Stretch?*

This exercise strengthens the core and the spine. A strong spine reduces your risk of vertebral fracture. This exercise also creates length in the spine by actively lengthening through each vertebra. Instead of shrinking, you'll be growing! (I've actually had clients who have grown half an inch after beginning an OsteoPilates program—it is a result of improved posture and an emphasis on lengthening).

### Reminders

For details, see the Reminder Glossary.

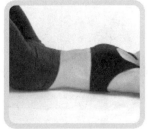

*Flat
Spine*

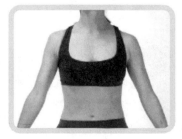

*Wide
Shoulders*

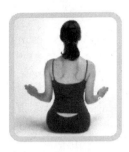

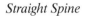

*Straight Spine*

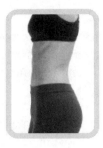

*Lifted Core*

**You don't want to look like this!**

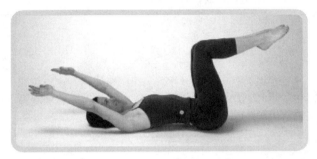

*Don't allow the spine to release. If your spine is released, the core can't work. Keep the core lifting and working. If you can't keep the legs straight, keep them as straight as you can so that the exercise becomes a stretch for the backs of the legs also.*

## Elbow Lifts

*Safe for low bone density*

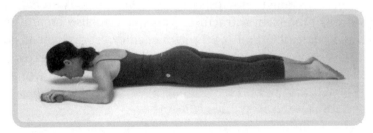

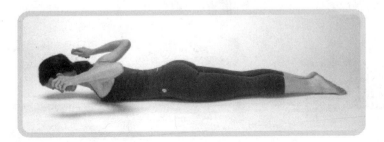

### Getting Started

Lie on your stomach with your arms bent and slightly out from your sides. Keep your core lifting and your legs squeezing together.

### Moving

Pinch the shoulder blades gently together and lift both arms off the floor. Don't allow the elbows to sag—they should be as high as the hands.

### Breathing

Exhale, lift the arms. Inhale, lower back down.

### Repetitions:   8–16.

### Keep This in Mind

Keep the shoulders pushing down your back and away from your ears. You can imagine that you are sliding your shoulders down into your hip pockets.

### Picture This

Imagine yourself on a medieval stretching rack. Keep your neck and spine long by reaching through the crown of your head in one direction and imagine the tailbone and legs being pulled in the other direction. This is an image you can use with every OsteoPilates exercise.

### Why Are We Doing *Elbow Lifts?*

This exercise is for strengthening the spine to promote good posture and to lower fracture risk. The lifting of the arms also stretches the front of the shoulders in order to release tension and to allow correct posture to be possible. It's hard to keep your shoulders pulled back if there are muscles that are constantly tugging them forward. Also, the active lengthening of the spine through the head and tailbone, as well as feeling long through the legs, elongates the spine and releases tension as well as puts more room between the vertebrae. Instead of feeling crunched, you'll feel long.

### Reminders

For details, see the Reminder Glossary.

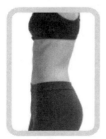
*Lifted Core*

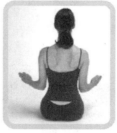
*Straight Spine*

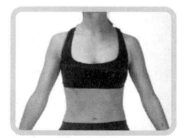
*Wide Shoulders*

**You don't want to look like this!**

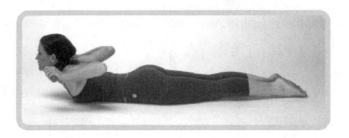

*Do not look up when you are performing Elbow Lifts. Allow the spine to be straight, long, and in alignment by looking down at the floor. Don't relax the core muscles or your low back will sag and feel crunched. Lift your core and elongate!*

# The Hundred I

*Safe for low bone density*

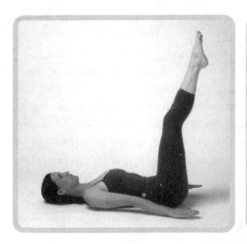 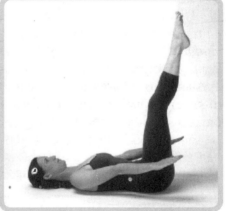

## Getting Started

Lying on your back, lift the arms 4 inches off the floor as you extend them past the hips. With the knees directly over the hips, straighten the legs toward the ceiling as much as you can.

### Moving

Begin rapidly and forcefully pumping your straight arms up and down in about a 4-inch range of motion. The pumps should be small, quick, and firm.

### Breathing

While you inhale, pump the arms five times. Exhale, pump five times.

**Repetitions:** 5–10 sets. One set is 10 pumps of the arms or one inhale and one exhale.

### Keep This in Mind

Keep the back pressed into the floor. Keep the arms straight and firm, not wobbly or flimsy. You should not feel stress in your neck and shoulders. If you do, you're working your stomach muscles too hard. Bend your knees a little bit and bring them toward your chest.

### Picture This

Elongate the spine by imagining that one strand of your hair is being pulled away and lengthening your spine along with it, like a puppet on a string.

### Why Are We Doing *The Hundred I?*

This exercise was created as a breathing exercise, as well as an abdominal exercise. Use *Breathing*, version B while you are performing *The Hundred I* (as well as *all* of these exercises). The core muscles and the arms are being strengthened. A strong core improves your ability to balance and, in turn, reduces your fracture risk. If your hamstrings are tight, this exercise will also promote flexibility, which can increase ease of movement and decrease back pain.

### Reminders

For details, see the Reminder Glossary.

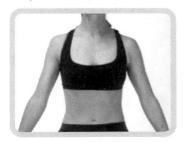
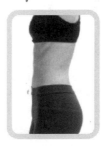
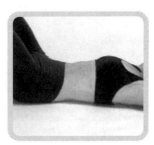

*Wide Shoulders*          *Lifted Core*          *Flat Spine*

**You don't want to look like this!**

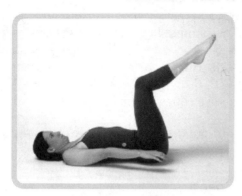

*Do not allow the back to pull away from the floor. Don't let the shoulders creep up to the ears. Keep the shoulders pressing down your back. Don't bend your knees any more than you need to. Keep the legs as straight as possible in order to stretch the hamstrings.*

# Leg Pull Back I

*Safe for low bone density*

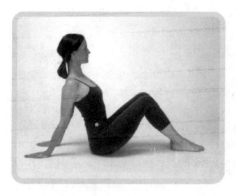 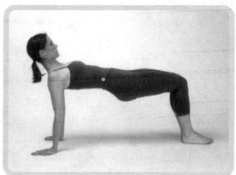

## Getting Started

Sit up straight with your feet hip-width apart and about a foot or so from your hips. Support your back with your hands behind your hips.

## Moving

Lift your hips off the floor and then return to a seated position.

## Challenge

After you have lifted the hips up, take one leg off the floor. Repeat with the other leg.

## Breathing

Exhale, lift up. Inhale, come back down.

**Repetitions:** 4–8.

### Keep This in Mind

Keep the spine straight and the stomach lifted while doing this exercise. Keep your shoulder blades gently pinching together. Press your shoulders down and away from your ears so that they don't creep up around your neck. Keep your weight evenly distributed between your hands and feet.

### Picture This

Imagine a little fire under your hips from which you have to keep lifting higher to get away from the heat.

### Why Are We Doing *Leg Pull Back I?*

This exercise strengthens the upper back, arms, stomach, and hips. All of these elements combined help to strengthen the muscles that create better posture and, therefore, help you to better avoid a flexed spine. Increased spine and core strength also reduces your risk of fracture. The pressure that you are placing on your hands will help to increase bone density at the wrist.

### Reminders

For details, see the Reminder Glossary.

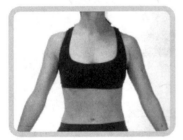
*Wide Shoulders*

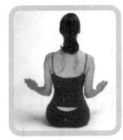
*Straight Spine*

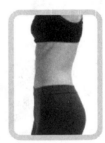
*Lifted Core*

**You don't want to look like this!**

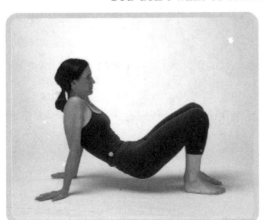

*Don't sink into your shoulders. Don't put all of your weight on your hands. Do not slouch or flex the spine.*

# Leg Pull Front I

*Safe for low bone density*

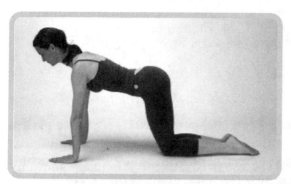

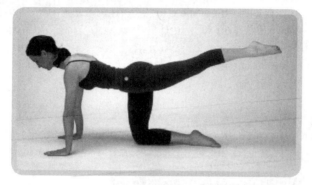

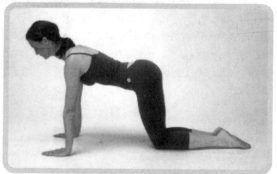

## Getting Started

Get down on your hands and knees. Do not let your low back sag, and do not allow your upper back to round. Keep the core lifted and the spine elongated.

## Moving

Stretch the right leg out behind you and then bring it back. Repeat with the left leg.

### Challenge

When your right leg is lifted, try taking your left arm off the floor. The arm should extend in front of you in the opposite direction of the leg.

### Breathing

Exhale, lift the leg. Inhale, bring it back in.

**Repetitions:** 4–8 on each side.

### Keep This in Mind

In order to put your spine in perfect alignment, have someone place a dowel or a yardstick along your spine. You should feel the back of your head, the space between the shoulder blades, and the tailbone touching the dowel. There should be a little bit of space under the dowel by the neck and the low back. You can check your alignment by using this method on many of the exercises. You will find that if you are able to achieve good alignment while on all fours, or when you are lying on your side, that it will be much easier to attain perfect alignment when you are standing or sitting.

### Picture This

Imagine that your torso is sandwiched between the ceiling and the floor. No sagging or arching will be possible.

### Why Are We Doing *Leg Pull Front I?*

Differently than sitting or standing, this exercise places focus on posture in an alignment that will improve your overall posture. Your shoulder, spine, core, and hamstring strength is also being increased. It is important to increase spine and core strength in order to improve your balance, which will reduce your risk of fracture.

### Reminders

For details, see the Reminder Glossary.

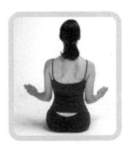

*Straight Spine*

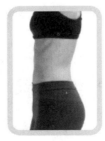

*Lifted Core*

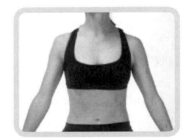

*Wide Shoulders*

**You don't want to look like this!**

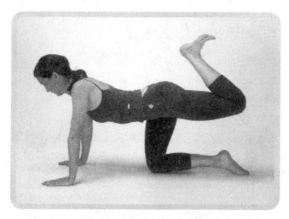

*Don't sag or arch the spine. Don't allow the chin to jut out—keep it tucked in. If your focus is anywhere but on the floor while you are doing this exercise, then check your alignment.*

# Mermaid

*Safe for low bone density*

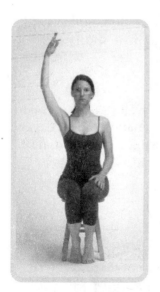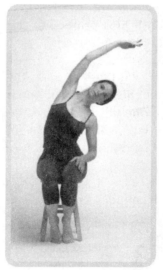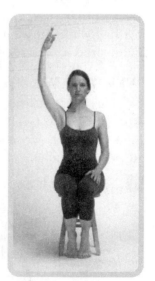

## Getting Started

Sitting on a firm chair, reach the right arm straight overhead. Be sure to keep the right shoulder pressing down as you reach the right hand toward the ceiling.

## Moving

Look straight ahead and begin side-bending. Keep the right hip firmly pressing down as your reach to the left.

## Challenge

Do this exercise while seated on the floor with the legs extended straight in front of you.

## Breathing

Inhale, reach to the ceiling. Exhale, side-bend. Inhale, pause in the side bend. Exhale, return to start.

**Repetitions:**   3–6 on each side.

## Keep This in Mind

Be sure to side-bend and to not twist the spine. You can imagine that a piece of plywood has been placed behind you and that you have to keep both shoulder blades on it for the entire exercise. Also, if you continue looking straight ahead and not at the floor, it will help to prevent you from twisting. Twisting defeats the purpose of the exercise, and it is also an osteoporosis no-no.

## Picture This

In order to increase your side-stretch, imagine side-bending over a big ball while pressing both hips firmly into the floor. If you have a medium-sized exercise ball, you can use it!

## Why Are We Doing *Mermaid?*

This exercise stretches the sides of the spine as well as increases core strength. Many of us have one side of our back that is tighter or less flexible than the other. *Mermaid* begins to even that imbalance out. So don't be surprised if, initially, you can't bend as far on one side as the other.

## Reminders

For details, see the Reminder Glossary.

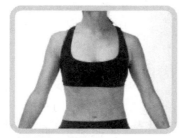

*Wide Shoulders*

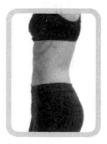

*Lifted Core*

**You don't want to look like this!**

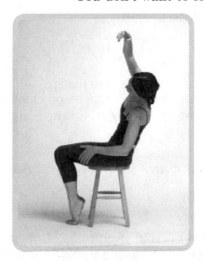

*Don't slouch forward. Don't twist. Keep the shoulder blades gently pinching together to help you keep the shoulders square.*

# Rowing

*Safe for low bone density*

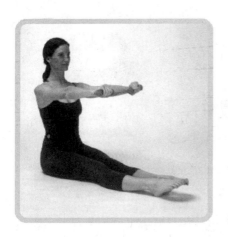 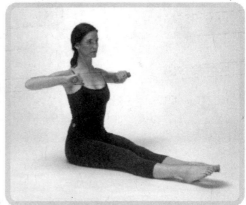

## Getting Started

Sit up straight with your legs extended out in front of you. Alternately, you can do this while seated in a chair if you can't get the spine straight while seated on the floor.

## Moving

Pinch your shoulder blades together and bring your hands toward the shoulders.

## Challenge

Add hand weights.

## Breathing

Inhale, row. Exhale, extend back to start.

## Repetitions: 8–16.

## Keep This in Mind

Be sure to sit up straight. Initiate the movement by pinching the shoulder blades together. Keep the shoulders dropped and the core lifted.

## Picture This

Imagine that you are rowing through thick molasses. Add pressure and resistance to the movement.

## Why Are We Doing *Rowing?*

This exercise will help to improve your posture by strengthening the muscles between the shoulder blades. Working the core muscles, while performing *Rowing,* will improve your balance and reduce your fracture risk.

## Reminders

For details, see the Reminder Glossary.

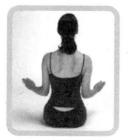
*Straight Spine*

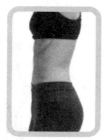
*Lifted Core*

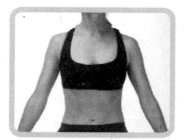
*Wide Shoulders*

### You don't want to look like this!

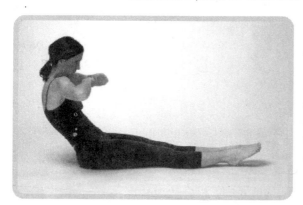

*Do not slouch or flex the spine. Do not jut the chin forward—keep it tucked in. Do not allow the stomach muscles to relax. Lift the core muscles.*

# Shoulder Stretch

*Safe for low bone density*

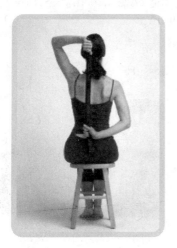 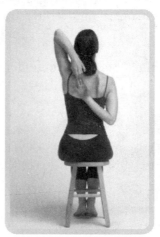

### Getting Started

Sit up straight. Put a towel in your right hand and drop the towel behind the right shoulder. Keep the right elbow back and almost out of your peripheral vision.

### Moving

Grab the bottom of the towel with your left hand. Walk the left hand up the towel, getting as close to the right hand as possible. Eventually, you may be able to walk the hands close enough together that you no longer need the towel.

### Breathing

Deeply inhale and exhale while you hold the stretch.

**Repetitions:** 90 seconds on each side.

### Keep This in Mind

Keep the spine straight. Only reach as far up on the towel as you can comfortably go—don't overstretch. If you can't hold the stretch for 90 seconds, you are overstretching.

### Picture This

Imagine that you are trying to scratch that hard-to-reach spot on your back, but that you are also sandwiched between two boards that give you no forward or backward movement.

### Why Are We Doing *Shoulder Stretch*?

Tight shoulder muscles can often prevent good posture. These tight muscles create a rounded or hunched upper back. Stretching them will make perfect posture easy. Lifting the core will make your abdominals and spine stronger and reduce fracture risk.

### Reminders

For details, see the Reminder Glossary.

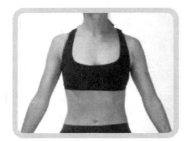
*Wide Shoulders*

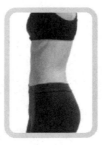
*Lifted Core*

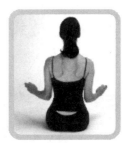
*Straight Spine*

**You don't want to look like this!**

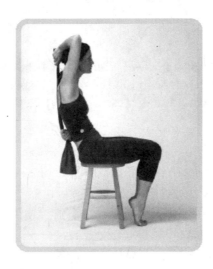

*Don't slouch. Don't relax the stomach muscles. Sit up straight and lift the core.*

# Shrugs

*Safe for low bone density*

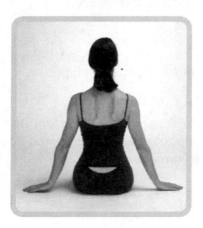

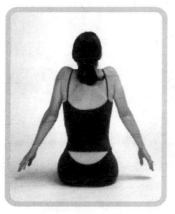 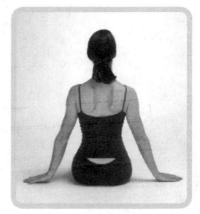

### Getting Started

Sit up straight in a chair or on the floor with the legs extended straight in front of you. Gently pinch the shoulder blades behind you.

### Moving

Vigorously press the shoulders down away from the ears. Relax. Now push the shoulders up to the ears.

### Challenge

Add hand weights, starting at about 2–3 pounds.

### Breathing

Inhale, press down. Exhale, shrug up.

**Repetitions:**    8–16.

### Keep This in Mind

Avoid the tendency to sink into the low back. Keep pressing the low back forward as you lift the core muscles. Be sure to create as large a range of motion with the shoulders as possible.

### Picture This

Imagine that you are a turtle and you are poking your head in and out of your shell. Be sure not to hunch the upper back.

### Why Are We Doing *Shrugs?*

Even though it feels like you are adding tension to the shoulders, this exercise can actually help to reduce shoulder and neck tension. Increased shoulder strength from this exercise can also help to reduce neck pain. This is a great exercise for anyone who spends a lot of time sitting. *Shrugs* improves posture by increasing strength in the muscles that support proper alignment.

### Reminders

For details, see the Reminder Glossary.

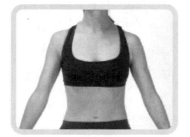 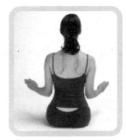 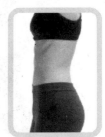

*Wide Shoulders*  *Straight Spine*  *Lifted Core*

**You don't want to look like this!**

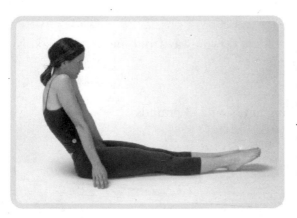

*Do not allow your spine to sink back. Sit up straight. Do not round your shoulders forward when you shrug up to your ears. Pinch the shoulder blades together.*

# Side Kicks I: Front/Back

*Safe for low bone density*

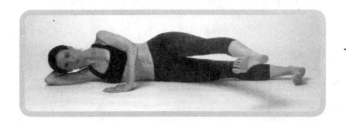

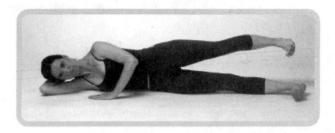

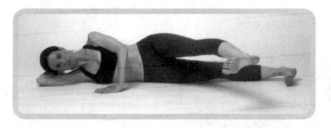

### Getting Started

Lie on your right side in a slight L shape. The legs should be slightly forward of your straight torso. Keep shoulder over shoulder and hip over hip.

### Moving

Lift the left leg about 4 inches. Flex the foot and swing it forward as far as you can while keeping the shoulders and hips from moving. At the end of the swing forward, give an extra little pulse or kick. Now swing the leg behind you and give two little kicks in the back.

### Challenge

Do the exercise without the support of the left hand. Keep the shoulders and hips still.

### Breathing

Inhale, swing forward. Exhale, swing back.

**Repetitions:** 8. Repeat with the other leg.

### Keep This in Mind

It is very important to keep the torso still on this exercise. A still torso makes the spine, core and leg muscles work. Otherwise, you are just swinging your leg around. Be aware that you will not be able to swing very far behind you while keeping the spine still. Keep your waist lifted off the mat while doing this exercise. Even if you can't slide your hand under your waist, that is the intention.

### Picture This

Imagine that you have placed a thin dowel from your shoulder to your hip. Don't let it fall off.

### Why Are We Doing *Side Kicks I Front/Back?*

This exercise strengthens the outsides of the legs, the spine, and core muscles, as well as improving coordination. Improved coordination helps to reduce fracture risk. Strong legs will make standing and walking much more effortless—you won't fatigue as easily.

### Reminders

For details, see the Reminder Glossary.

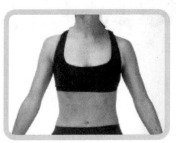
*Wide Shoulders*

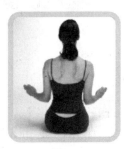
*Straight Spine*

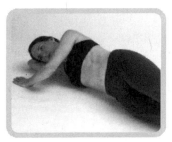
*Hip Over Hip...*

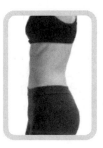
*Lifted Core*

**You don't want to look like this!**

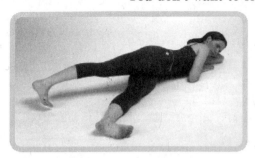

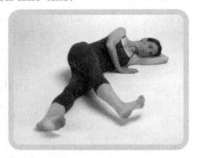

*Do not roll the torso and hips forward when the leg goes back.*

*Do not roll the hips and torso back when the leg kicks forward.*

# Side Kicks II: Small Circles

*Safe for low bone density*

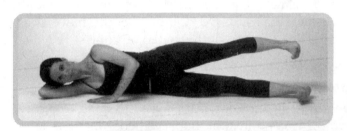

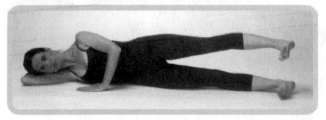

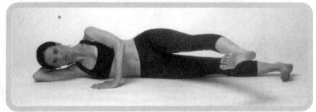

### Getting Started

Lie on your right side in a slight L shape. The legs should be slightly forward of your straight torso. Keep shoulder over shoulder and hip over hip.

### Moving

Flex the left foot and make small, 8- to 10-inch circles with the top leg.

### Challenge

Take the left hand off the floor to make your core and spine work harder.

### Breathing

Inhale for two circles. Exhale for two circles.

**Repetitions:**  8–16 in each direction. Repeat with the other leg.

### Keep This in Mind

Keep the toes facing straight in front of you instead of even slightly toward the ceiling, and you will keep the work at the hip. If you turn the toes to the ceiling you will be working the front of the leg a little bit more. Either way is fine. Try alternating. Lift the waist off the floor. Even if you can't slide your hand under your waist while doing this exercise, that is the intention.

### Picture This

Imagine that you are lying next to a wall and that your hips and shoulders are just slightly brushing against it. Don't allow them to move away or press into the wall. You don't have to just imagine this one—try it and see if you can do it!

### Why Are We Doing *Side Kicks II: Small Circles?*

This exercise strengthens the outsides of the legs, the spine, and core muscles, as well as improving coordination. Improved coordination helps to reduce fracture risk. Strong legs will make standing and walking much more effortless—you won't fatigue as easily.

### Reminders

For details, see the Reminder Glossary.

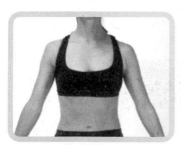

Wide
Shoulders

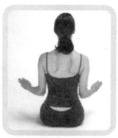

Straight
Spine

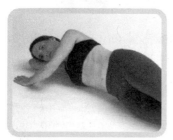

Hip Over Hip...

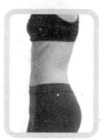

Lifted Core

**You don't want to look like this!**

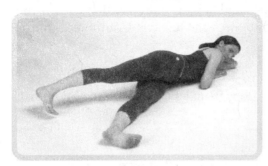
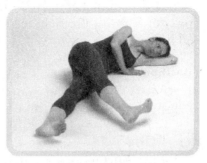

*Do not roll the torso and hips forward when the leg goes back.*

*Do not roll the hips and torso back when the leg kicks forward.*

# Side Kicks III: Lower Leg Lift

*Safe for low bone density*

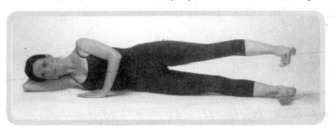

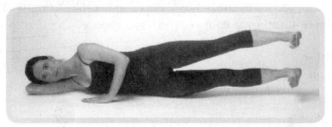

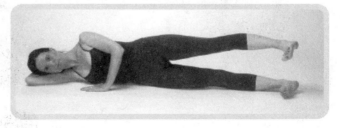

### Getting Started

Lie on your right side in a slight L shape. The legs should be slightly forward of your straight torso. Keep shoulder over shoulder and hip over hip.

### Moving

Lift the left leg about 4-8 inches and keep it there, stationary, for this exercise. Now lift the right leg up to meet the left leg. Continue to lift up and down.

### Challenge

Remove the left hand from the floor to make the spine and abdominals work harder.

### Breathing

Inhale, lift the right leg. Exhale, lower it back down.

**Repetitions:** 8. Repeat with the other leg.

### Keep This in Mind

Don't roll the hips back as you lift the bottom leg. It is easy to allow the feet to get into weird shapes on this exercise. Keep the feet flexed and pointing straight ahead. Keep your waist lifted off the mat. Even if you can't slide your hand under your waist, that is the intention.

### Picture This

Imagine that your feet are pressing against a flat surface. You can feel your big toe, little toe, and heel all pushing equally against the surface.

### Why Are We Doing *Side Kicks III: Lower Leg Lift?*

This exercise increases inner thigh, core, and spine strength. All of these improvements will improve your balance and reduce your fracture risk.

### Reminders

For details, see the Reminder Glossary.

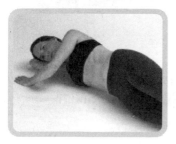
*Wide Shoulders*

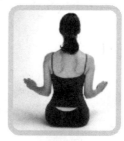
*Straight Spine*

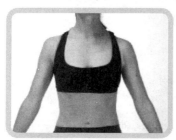
*Hip Over Hip...*

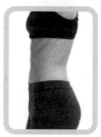
*Lifted Core*

**You don't want to look like this!**

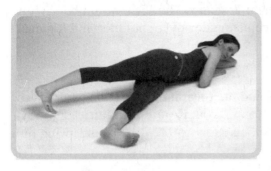 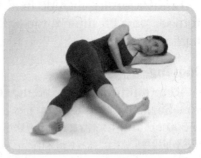

*Do not roll the torso and hips forward or back as you lift the leg up and down.*

# Side Kicks IV: Rotations

*Safe for low bone density*

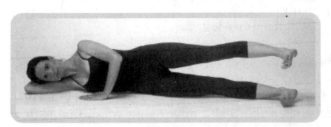

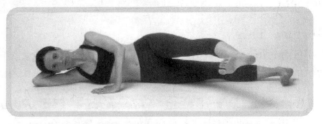

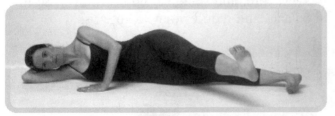

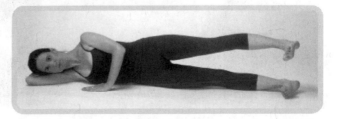

### Getting Started

Lie on your right side in a slight L shape. The legs should be slightly forward of your straight torso. Keep shoulder over shoulder and hip over hip.

### Moving

The left foot should be flexed and the toes should be facing in front of you. Swing it about 8-10 inches in front of you. Rotate the entire leg so that the knee and toe are facing the ceiling. Now rotate it back and swing the leg back to your start position.

### Challenge

Remove the left hand from the floor to make the spine and abdominals work harder.

### Breathing

Inhale, swing the leg forward. Exhale, rotate the leg. Inhale, "un-rotate" the leg. Exhale, bring the leg back to start.

**Repetitions:** 8. Repeat with the other leg.

### Keep This in Mind

You should feel the leg rotating from the hip. The movement of the knee and foot are just a result of the hip motion. Keep your waist lifted off the floor. Even if you can't slide your hand under your waist, that is the intention.

### Picture This

Imagine that your working leg is lying under a trapdoor. Imagine that your foot is pushing the trapdoor open and then allowing it close again.

### Why Are We Doing *Side Kicks IV: Rotations?*

This exercise increases leg, core, and spine strength. All of these increases will improve your balance and reduce your fracture risk.

### Reminders

For details, see the Reminder Glossary.

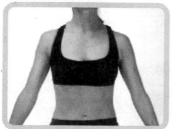
*Wide Shoulders*

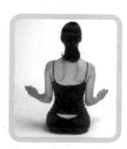
*Straight Spine*

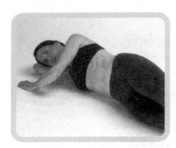

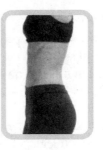

*Hip Over Hip...*          *Lifted Core*

**You don't want to look like this!**

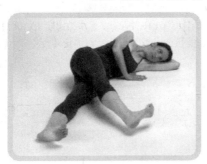

*Do not roll the hips and torso back when the leg moves forward and rotates.*

# Single Leg Kick

*Safe for low bone density*

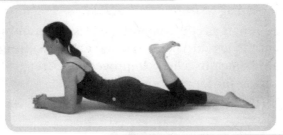

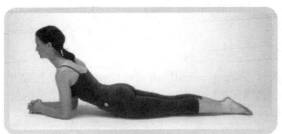

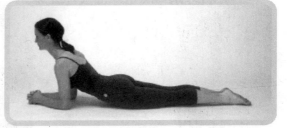

### Getting Started

Lying on your stomach, prop yourself up on your elbows with your hands clasped in front of you. Lift the stomach away from the floor and toward the spine. Legs are lengthened away from your hips and squeezed together.

### Moving

Bend the left knee and give a quick double kick, or pump, toward the hips. Now lengthen the left leg back down onto the mat. Repeat on the right side.

### Challenge

Lift the working leg 1 inch above the mat. Keep a 1-inch space under the thigh as you double pump the leg. Be sure to keep the legs squeezing together—don't turn out.

### Breathing

Exhale as you double pump the leg. Inhale, lengthen back to your start position.

**Repetitions:** 8 on each side.

### Keep This in Mind

When you bring the heel toward the hip, both knees should still be touching. Do not allow the foot of the moving leg to drift across center and toward your other hip. Keep your shoulders pressing down and away from your ears. Maintain a long spine.

### Picture This

Imagine that you are a seal balancing a ball on the top of your head. You are also trying to get the ball closer to the ceiling. Stretch and pull your spine long toward the ceiling.

### Why Are We Doing *Single Leg Kick*?

This exercise strengthens the backs of the legs, core, and spine muscles. While the backs of the legs are being strengthened, the fronts of the legs, or quadriceps, are being stretched. Improved leg strength will give you more stamina walking for long periods of time.

### Reminders

For details, see the Reminder Glossary.

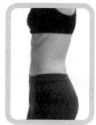

*Lifted Core*

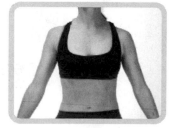

*Wide Shoulders*

**You don't want to look like this!**

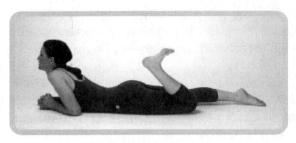

*Don't relax into your shoulders. Push the shoulders down. Don't sink into your waist. Lift all the core muscles. Don't allow the legs to come apart—keep them together.*

# Single Leg Stretch I

*Safe for low bone density*

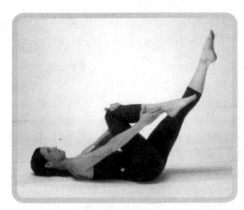

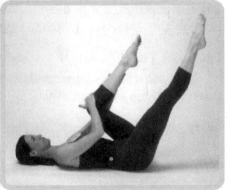

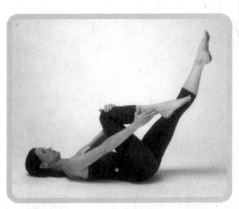

### Getting Started

Lie flat on your back. Put the left hand on the right knee, and the right hand on the right ankle. The left leg extends toward the ceiling. Lower the left leg just enough to feel moderate pressure on the abdominals.

### Moving

Switch legs. Hug the left knee in with the right hand on the left knee, and the left hand on the left ankle. Now, switch again. You'll notice that in the second photo, the leg that is bent is higher than the previous photo. Bring the leg to wherever you are most comfortable. If the knees are a little glitchy, don't bend them quite as much.

### Challenge

Keep lowering the extended leg to add more and more abdominal work.

### Breathing

Inhale for two changes and exhale for two changes

**Repetitions:** 8–16 changes.

### Keep This in Mind

This is a very active exercise. Even when you are hugging one knee in, that same knee is trying to push away from the hand. The hand that is touching the ankle is pushing into the ankle as the ankle pushes into the hand. Keep the energy moving. Avoid the tendency to round the shoulders on this exercise by opening the shoulders flat on the floor.

### Picture This

Imagine a mass of energy that circles from the chest, through the arms, down the thigh of the bent leg, up the stomach, and back to the chest.

### Why Are We Doing *Single Leg Stretch P.*

This exercise increases levels of coordination while strengthening the core, spine, and leg muscles. Scientists have proven that individuals with strong back muscles are less likely to fracture.

### Reminders

For details, see the Reminder Glossary.

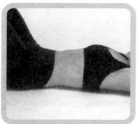
*Flat Spine*

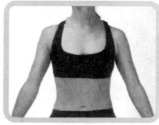
*Wide Shoulders*

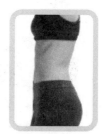
*Lifted Core*

**You don't want to look like this!**

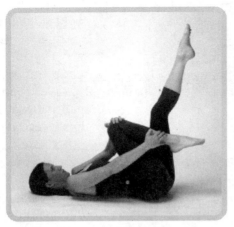

*Don't release the spine from the floor. If your spine is releasing and your stomach muscles are protruding, then you are lowering the extended leg too much. Don't round the shoulders. Keep them flat and wide.*

# Stretches

*Safe for low bone density*

### Low Back Stretch

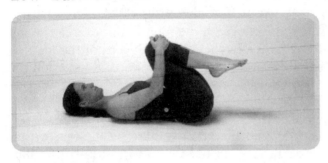

Lie on your back and hug your knees to your chest.

### Hamstring Stretch

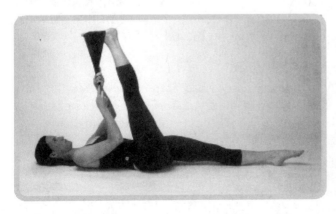

Lie on your back and hug the left knee into your chest. Wrap a towel around the arch of that foot. Straighten the leg as much as you can. If you can straighten it, pull the leg toward you. Keep the back of the right thigh pressing toward the floor. Repeat on the other side.

### Quadricep Stretch

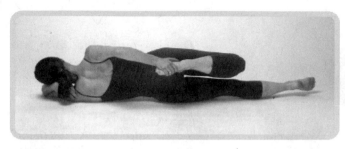

Lie on your right side and bend your left foot toward your hips. Grab the foot with your left hand and pull it toward your hips. Repeat on the other side.

### Breathing

Breathe deeply while holding the stretches.

**Repetitions:** 90 seconds each.

### Keep This in Mind

**Low Back Stretch:** Do not allow the chin to jut toward the ceiling. Keep the chin tucked in and pulling actively toward the back of the neck.

**Hamstring Stretch:** If you are having trouble straightening the leg, don't worry. Keep practicing—your flexibility will increase rapidly.

**Quadriceps Stretch:** If you can't reach the foot on this exercise, don't worry. The hamstring stretch also stretches the quadriceps of the leg that is lying on the floor. Just keep pushing it into the floor. Soon you'll be flexible enough to do this version also.

### Picture This

Whenever you do a stretch, imagine that you are pushing in two directions. For the low back stretch, pull the thighs in and push the hips down. For the hamstring stretch, pull the towel leg in, push the hips down, and push the floor leg actively into the floor. For the quadriceps stretch, pull the foot toward the hip and try stretching the knee of that same leg toward the foot of the leg that is lying on the floor.

### Why Are We Doing *Stretches?*

Increased flexibility equals increased ease of movement. Studies have shown that increased flexibility will help you to increase your strength. Low back flexibility decreases low back pain. Increased hamstring flexibility will allow you to do more activities without flexing the spine (an osteoporosis no-no) as well as decrease back pain. Quadricep flexibility can also decrease back pain, as well help to improve your posture and lend an ease of movement to all that you do.

## Reminders

For details, see the Reminder Glossary.

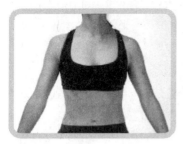
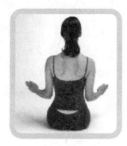
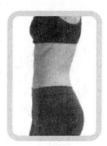

*Wide Shoulders*          *Straight Spine*          *Lifted Core*

# Swan I

*Safe for low bone density*

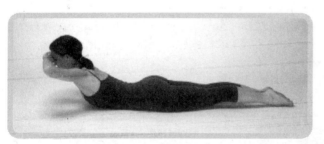

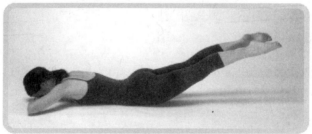

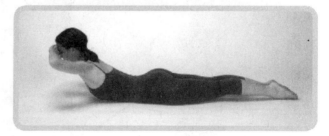

## Getting Started

Lie on your stomach with your forehead placed on your hands. Squeeze your legs together and lift your waist toward the spine.

167

### Moving

Keeping your forehead on your hands, lift the head, shoulders, and arms off the floor. As the upper body lowers back down, lift the legs off the floor. Now, lower your legs and lift your upper body.

### Challenge

Extend your arms over your head while you perform this exercise.

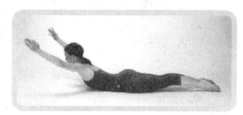

### Breathe

Inhale, lift the chest. Exhale, lift the legs.

### Repetitions: 6–10.

### Keep This in Mind

Keep the neck and head in line with the spine. Don't look up and put a crook in the neck. Keep your legs very straight. Your feet won't go as high but you'll be working harder. As an additional note of interest here, this exercise never gets any easier. As you get stronger you just go higher. It's always challenging.

### Picture This

Imagine that you are a teeter-totter or seesaw. As one half of you goes down the other half goes up.

### Why Are We Doing *Swan I?*

Spine strength is very important for posture, back health, and reduced fracture risk. The back muscles are often overlooked in favor of abdominal exercises. For someone with low bone density, spine strength is crucial for lowering fracture risk and preventing a flexed spine position.

### Reminders

For details, see the Reminder Glossary.

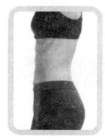

*Lifted Core*

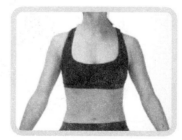

*Wide Shoulders*

**You don't want to look like this!**

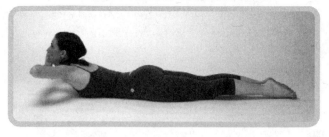

*Don't look up or take the head off the hands. Keep the spine long. Squeeze the legs together and don't bend the knees. Point your feet for added length and stretch in the legs.*

# Swan II

*Safe for low bone density*

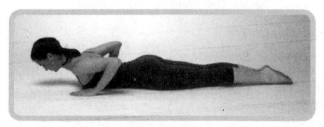

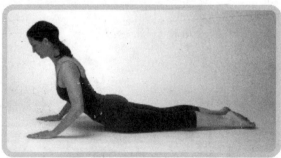

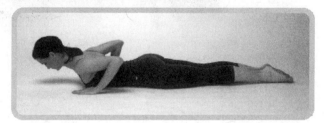

## Getting Started

Lie on your stomach with your hands under your shoulders and your stomach lifted away from the floor.

### Moving

Very slowly, begin to straighten the arms in order to lift the torso away from the mat. Be sure to continue lifting the stomach toward the spine. Now lower back to the mat.

### Breathing

Inhale, lift the spine. Exhale, lower back down.

### Repetitions: 4–8.

### Keep This in Mind

Press the shoulders away from the ears. Keep the spine long. The head and neck should just be going along for a ride on top of the spine. Don't look up and put a crink between the neck and the spine.

### Picture This

Imagine that you are creating an arc with your spine. Your feet are point A, which doesn't move. Your head is point B, which lifts, lengthens, and changes the shape of the line for the longest possible arc.

### Why Are We Doing *Swan II?*

This exercise increases spine flexibility and strength. The increased pressure through the arms will help to increase bone density at the wrist. Keep lifting the core muscles and you will improve your abdominal strength as well as your balance.

### Reminders

For details, see the Reminder Glossary.

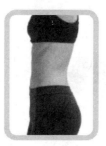
*Lifted Core*

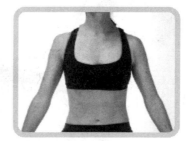
*Wide Shoulders*

**You don't want to look like this!**

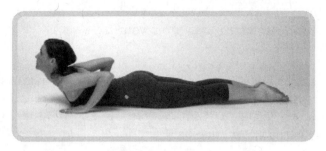

*Don't look up with the chin. Don't let the shoulders relax and push up to the ears. Don't allow the stomach to sag into the mat.*

# Swimming

*Safe for low bone density*

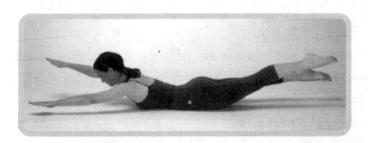

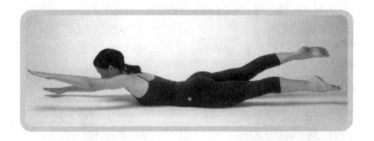

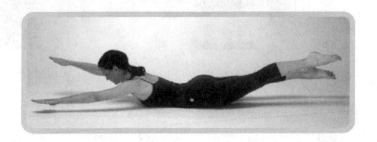

### Getting Started

Lie on your stomach with your arms extended overhead. Your legs are together and stretching away from your hips.

### Moving

Lift the upper body and legs off the floor. Lift the right arm and left leg a little higher. Leaving the body lifted for the entire exercise, lower the right arm and left leg and lift the left arm and right leg. Pick up the speed and continue alternating back and forth while staying lifted.

### Breathing

Inhale for four changes. Exhale for four changes.

**Repetitions:** 4–8 sets of 8 changes.

### Keep This in Mind

Pull the stomach toward the spine and keep the core lifted. Elongate the spine by stretching the arms and legs away from each other. Don't overthink this exercise. It is just a fluttering motion with arms and legs.

### Picture This

You are swimming! Imagine that you are floating on top of the water (your mat) and that your feet and hands are just splashing the top of the water.

### Why Are We Doing *Swimming?*

This exercise strengthens the back muscles to promote proper posture and to reduce fracture risk. This exercise also works on coordination, which reduces the risk of falling.

### Reminders

For details, see the Reminder Glossary.

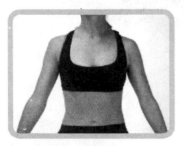

*Wide Shoulders*

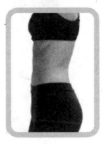

*Lifted Core*

**You don't want to look like this!**

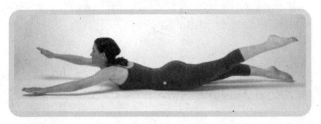

*Don't look up. Keep the spine long. Don't relax the core muscles. Keep lifting. Don't bend the arms and legs—keep them straight.*

# Toe Touches

*Safe for low bone density*

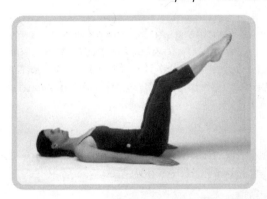

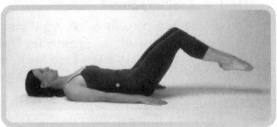

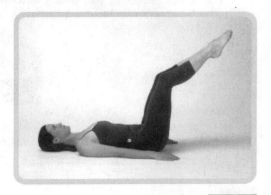

### Getting Started

Lie on your back with your knees directly over your hips. Extend the lower legs slightly above the knees.

### Moving

Keeping your spine pressed to the floor, arc the toes slightly away from the hips and toward the floor.

### Challenge

Eventually, reach your toes all the way to the floor with the spine pressed flat.

### Breathing

Exhale, lower the legs. Inhale, bring them back up.

### Repetitions: 4–12.

### Keep This in Mind

If you lower the legs to the point that the spine begins to release from the floor, then the abdominals are no longer working effectively. Keep the abdominals working by keeping the spine pressed flat. Don't worry about how low you are going. Your abdominals will gain strength only if you are working properly.

### Picture This

Imagine that you are drawing the arc of a rainbow with your toes. Don't just drop your toes straight down next to your hips.

### Why Are We Doing *Toe Touches?*

This exercise strengthens the core muscles, which are important for improving balance, improving posture, and reducing fracture risk. The fronts of the legs, or quadriceps, are also working hard, which will make them stronger for long walks and long periods of time spent on your feet.

### Reminders

For details, see the Reminder Glossary.

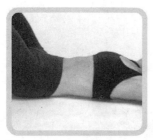
*Flat Spine*

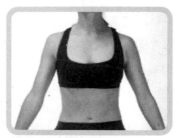
*Wide Shoulders*

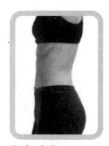
*Lifted Core*

**You don't want to look like this!**

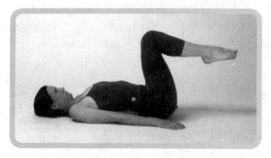

*Don't allow your spine to pull away from the mat. Don't drop your feet to the mat—arc them out and down. Don't bend your knees too much.*

# Wrist Presses

*Safe for low bone density*

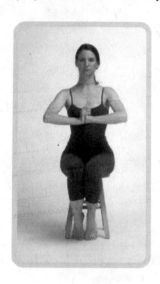

### Getting Started

Sitting in a chair or on the floor with the legs extended out in front of you, press the heels of the hands together.

### Moving

Press the heels of the hands together for 5 seconds and then release. Repeat.

### Breathing

Exhale, press. Inhale, release.

**Repetitions:** 6–12.

### Keep This in Mind.

Keep your spine straight. Don't slouch forward when you press the hands together. This is an isometric exercise. Provide yourself with enough resistance to "feel" the exercise, but don't make yourself suffer.

### Picture This

Imagine that you are pressing the thinnest piece of paper between your hands. If you relax at all, it will fall.

### Why Are We Doing *Wrist Presses?*

This exercise puts pressure on the wrists and encourages increased bone density at this site. Keep lifting the core while you perform this exercise and you will be strengthening the abdominals and spine, as well as reducing your risk of fracture.

### Reminders:

For details, see the Reminder Glossary.

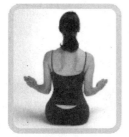
*Straight Spine*

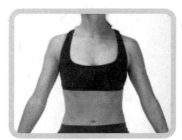
*Wide Shoulders*

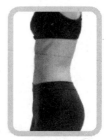
*Lifted Core*

**You don't want to look like this!**

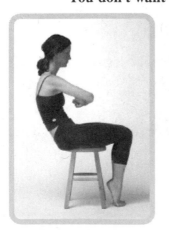

*Don't slouch forward. Don't allow the shoulders to round. Gently pinch the shoulder blades behind you as you do this exercise.*

# Exercise Programs

The following exercises have been put together to form complete programs. They progress from beginning to advanced. Even if you have a lot of exercise experience, start with the beginning program. Pilates exercises rely on specifics that you will learn in the first level and incorporate into the more advanced exercises.

## #1 Beginning Program for Low Bone Density

### Breathing

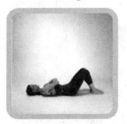

*Page 123*

### Toe Touches

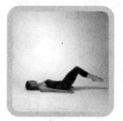

*Page 173*

### Bridging

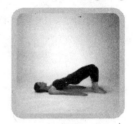

*Page 125*

### The Hundred I

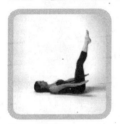

*Page 139*

### Low Back Stretch

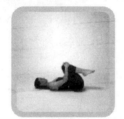

*Page 165*

### Puppet

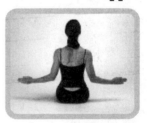

*Page 129*

### Chest Lifts

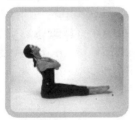

*Page 127*

### Shrugs

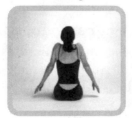

*Page 151*

### Wrist Presses

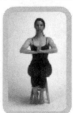

*Page 175*

### Rowing

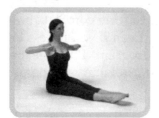

*Page 147*

### Shoulder Stretch

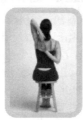

*Page 149*

### Side Kicks I

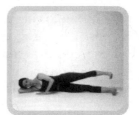

*Page 153*

### Hamstring Stretch

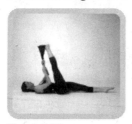

*Page 165*

### Swan I

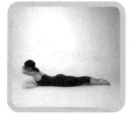

*Page 167*

### Elbow Lifts

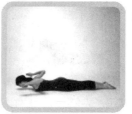

*Page 137*

### Balance

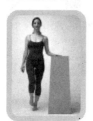

*Page 121*

## #2 Intermediate Program for Low Bone Density

This program contains several similarities to the first program. As you get stronger, we are not going to exclude all of the beginning exercises. Instead, we will just be adding more. I also recommend alternating programs 1 and 2.

### Breathing

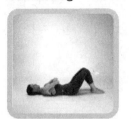

*Page 123*

### Toe Touches

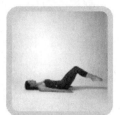

*Page 173*

### Bridging

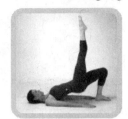

*Page 125*

### The Hundred I

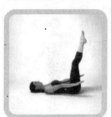

*Page 139*

### Single Leg Stretch I

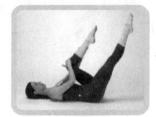

*Page 163*

### Chest Lifts

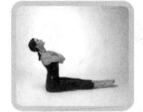

*Page 127*

### Diamonds

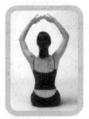

*Page 131*

### Puppet

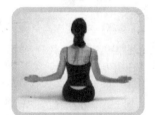

*Page 129*

### Wrist Presses

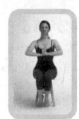

*Page 175*

### Mermaid

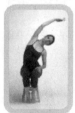

*Page 145*

### Side Kicks I

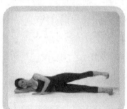

*Page 153*

### Side Kicks II

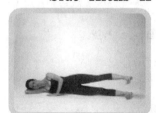

*Page 155*

**Quadricep Stretch**

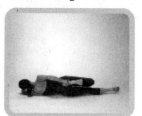

*Page 166*

**Swan I**

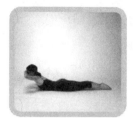

*Page 167*

**Single Leg Kick**

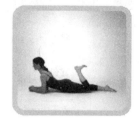

*Page 161*

**Double Leg Kick**

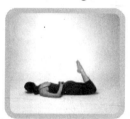

*Page 133*

**Shoulder Stretch**

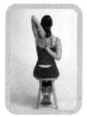

*Page 149*

**Balance**

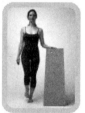

*Page 121*

## #3 Advanced Program for Low Bone Density

This is the advanced program and is not meant to be done before you can easily and competently complete programs 1 and 2. There are exercises in the beginning and intermediate programs that have been preparing you for this advanced program and should not be skipped. Once beginning program 3, I recommend alternating between the three programs.

Remember, the pictures here are only meant as reminders of the exercises elaborated on previously. Refer back to these descriptions to learn the specifics of all these exercises. Add the challenges to all of these exercises when you are ready.

**Breathing**

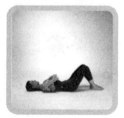

*Page 123*

**Toe Touches**

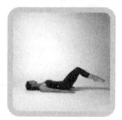

*Page 173*

**Bridging**

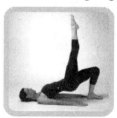

*Page 125*

**The Hundred I**

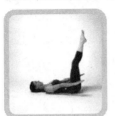

*Page 139*

**Single Leg Stretch I**

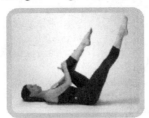

*Page 163*

**Double Leg Stretch**

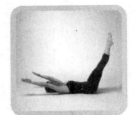

*Page 135*

**Puppet**

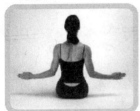

*Page 129*

**Rowing**

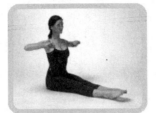

*Page 147*

**Mermaid**

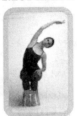

*Page 145*

**Quadricep Stretch**

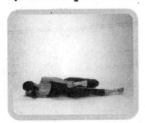

*Page 166*

**Side Kicks I**

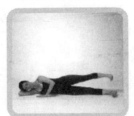

*Page 153*

**Side Kicks II**

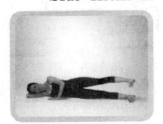

*Page 155*

**Side Kicks III**

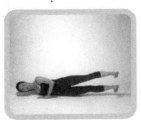

*Page 157*

**Side Kicks IV**

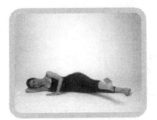

*Page 159*

**Hamstring Stretch**

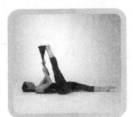

*Page 165*

### Quadricep Stretch

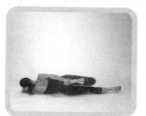

*Page 166*

### Swan I

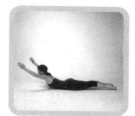

*Page 167*

### Swan II

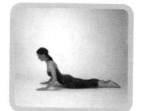

*Page 169*

### Swimming

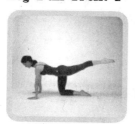

*Page 171*

### Single Leg Kick

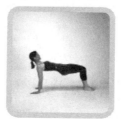

*Page 161*

### Double Leg Kick

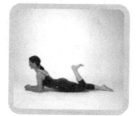

*Page 133*

### Leg Pull Front I

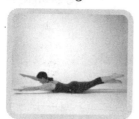

*Page 143*

### Leg Pull Back I

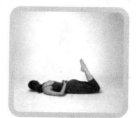

*Page 141*

### Shoulder Stretch

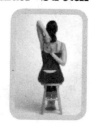

*Page 149*

### Balance

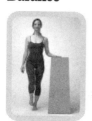

*Page 121*

# Chapter 8

## OsteoPilates:
### *Exercise Programs for Those With Normal Bone Density Only*

## Corkscrew

*For those with normal bone density only*

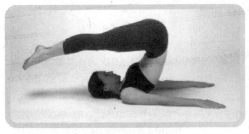
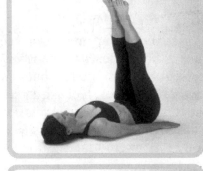
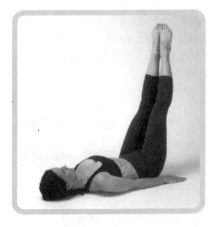
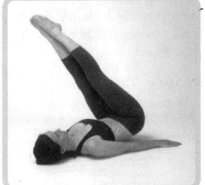

### Getting Started

Lying on your back, begin in the *Rollover* position (see the exercise called *Rollover* on page 200). Arms reach past the hips and your spine presses into the floor.

### Moving

Roll down the right side of your spine. Once your right hip is down, bring both hips down and your legs lower a little bit more. Now, shift your weight to the left and roll up the left side of your spine. Return to your start position.

### Breathing

Inhale, drop the legs right and center. Exhale, bring the legs left and center.

**Repetitions:**   4 in each direction.

### Let's Make This a Little Easier

Instead of beginning in the rollover position, just extend both legs straight up to the ceiling as you lie on your back. Drop both legs to the right. Then pass directly to a position that is center, but in which the legs are slightly lowered toward the floor. Now bring them up to the left (so that the position mirrors the first drop to the right) and then back to your start position with the legs extended up at center. Reverse direction after each one. Repeat 6 times in each direction.

### Keep This in Mind

As you roll up and down, keep your spine straight and don't allow the hips to creep closer to the ribcage. The same amount of space should be present between the hipbones and ribs as if you were standing. This exercise should almost feel like a massage for your back because you are rolling up and down on the muscles, not on the vertebrae. Keep your abdominals flat and pulled toward your spine. If your stomach muscles start to "pooch," you have lowered the legs too far.

Keep the legs firm and straight. You should feel the thigh muscles pulling up and away from your knees. If you are doing the modified version of this exercise with bent knees, imagine drawing circles on the ceiling with your knees.

### Picture This

Imagine that you are tracing the opening of an oval barrel with both feet. If the barrel is 6 inches off center to the right, be sure to drop 6 inches off center to the left.

## Reminders

For details, see the Reminder Glossary.

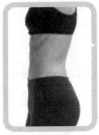
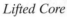
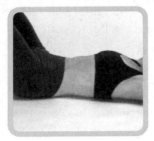
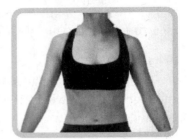

*Lifted Core*          *Flat Spine*          *Wide Shoulders*

# Double Leg Stretch II

*For those with normal bone density only*

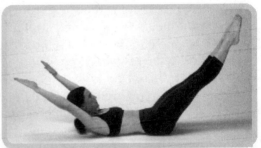

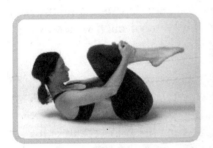
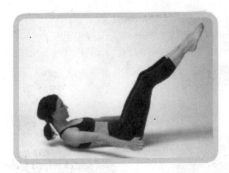
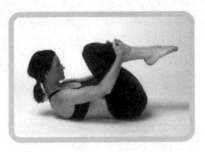

## Getting Started

Lie on your back and hug your knees to your chest to create a C-shaped spine. Try to touch your nose to your knees. Keep the head and shoulders lifted for the entire exercise.

## Moving

Extend the arms and legs to the ceiling. Lower the arms and legs away from each other while keeping the head and shoulders lifted. Now swing the arms wide and hug your knees back into your chest.

## Breathing

Inhale, extend the arms and legs to the ceiling. Exhale, lower the arms and legs. Inhale, swing the arms wide. Exhale, hug the knees in your start position.

**Repetitions:**   4–8.

## Challenge

Use small hand weights while performing this exercise.

## Keep This in Mind

Do not let the spine release from the floor. Only lower the legs as far as you can while keeping the spine from changing shape. Also, imagine the crown of the head and tailbone stretching away from each other in the longest C shape possible to keep the spine lengthening.

## Picture This

Imagine that you are holding a ball between your arms and legs. Now picture that ball getting bigger and bigger and pushing your arms overhead and toward the floor and your legs low and toward the floor. Your spine is still curved in a C shape around the ball for the entire exercise.

## Reminders

For details, see the Reminder Glossary.

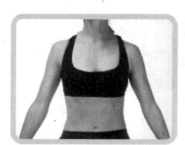
*Wide Shoulders*

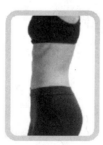
*Lifted Core*

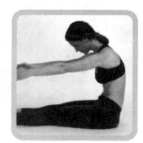
*C-shaped Spine*

# The Hundred II

*For those with normal bone density only*

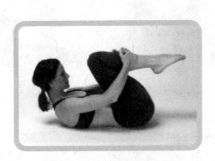 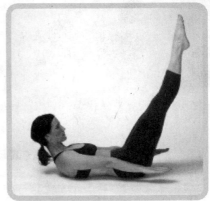

### Getting Started

Lie on your back with your legs hugged into your chest. Now, extend your legs up to the ceiling. Lower your legs until you feel tension in your stomach, but do not allow the spine to release from the mat. Lift your head and shoulders off the mat while you reach your arms long past your hips.

### Moving

Pump your arms up and down, in a 4- to 6-inch range, without moving your head and shoulders.

### Breathing

Exhale for 5 pumps of the arms. Inhale for 5 pumps.

**Repetitions:** 10 sets. One set is 10 pumps of the arms, or one exhale and one inhale.

### Challenge

Use small hand weights while your perform this exercise.

### Keep This in Mind

Keep your abdominals flat and pulled toward your spine. Do not allow your stomach to pooch out. If your legs are too low for your strength, your stomach will not be able to remain flat. If it is uncomfortable to do this exercise with straight legs, just bend the knees a little bit. Also, do not allow your head and shoulders to pump up and down—only the arms are pumping.

### Picture This

Imagine that you have spongy softballs under each upper arm. Now push down onto the balls rapidly and firmly as you pulse the arms.

### Reminders

For details, see the Reminder Glossary.

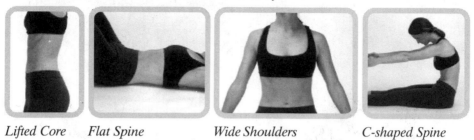

*Lifted Core*   *Flat Spine*        *Wide Shoulders*        *C-shaped Spine*

# Jackknife

*For those with normal bone density only*

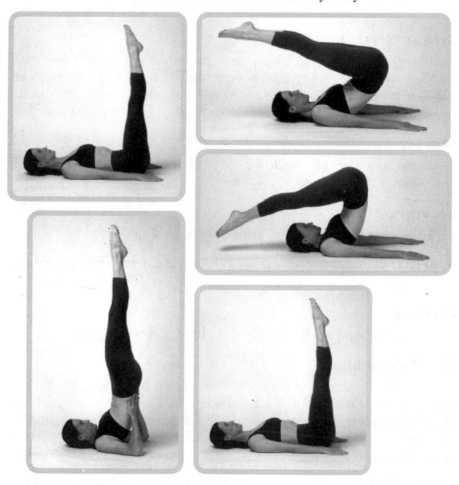

### Getting Started

Lie on your back with your legs extended to the ceiling. Each vertebra is pulled flat and your arms are pressing into the floor.

### Moving

Pull your lowest abdominal muscles (about 4 inches below your bellybutton) toward your spine and allow your feet to go over your head. Once overhead, extend your legs toward the ceiling. To get the legs as straight as possible, push your hips forward as your feet counterbalance by pushing back.

Bring your legs back down and roll back down through each vertebra until your feet are directly over your hips again.

### Breathing

Exhale, legs go overhead. Inhale, jackknife up. Exhale, lower back down. Inhale, pause. Exhale, roll down. Inhale, pause.

### Repetitions:  4–6.

### Challenge

Do not use your hands for support as you take your legs toward the ceiling. You won't go as high initially, but your abdominals will be working harder.

### Keep This in Mind

Be sure to initiate this exercise by squeezing the lowest abdominal muscles. As you continue to take the legs overhead, squeeze a little higher on the abdominals without allowing the lower abdominals to release. Keep squeezing a little higher and a little higher as those abdominals leave the floor. By the time your legs are completely overhead your entire abdominal region should be firm and pulled back. As you lift your straight legs toward the ceiling, keep the abdominals working and your arms pressing. Counterbalance with your hips and feet to get as high as possible.

### Picture This

Anytime you are working through the abdominals, imagine that you are a belly dancer. You are going to roll through the abdominals, beginning with the lowest abdominals when you are rolling down, or the highest abdominals if you are rolling up. Keep each abdominal group pulled to the spine as you recruit the next abdominal group.

### Reminders

For details, see the Reminder Glossary.

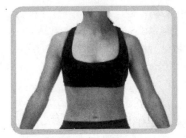
*Wide Shoulders*

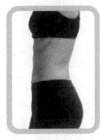
*Lifted Core*

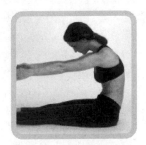
*C-shaped Spine*

# Jumping

*For those with normal bone density only*

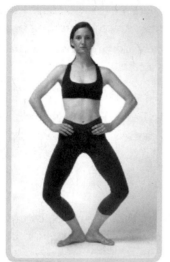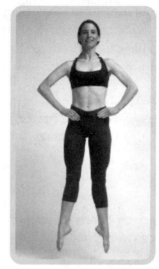

### Getting Started

Stand with your hands on your hips, heels together, and toes pointing slightly open and to the sides. Your knees should be facing over your toes so that when you bend your knees they point in the same direction as your feet.

### Moving

Bend your knees as deeply as you can *without* allowing the heels to leave the floor or the torso to lean forward. Now jump by pushing off with your feet. Your goal is to eventually push hard enough that your feet will be able to point in the air. When you land, land on the balls of the feet first, and roll through to the heels. Bend the knees immediately upon landing.

### Breathing

Inhale as you jump. Exhale as you land.

### Repetitions: 8–32.

### Keep This in Mind

You want to land as softly as possible when jumping—do not land with straight knees. Maintain perfect alignment through the spine and legs. When you jump, do not "buck" or throw the shoulders back behind your hips. When you land be sure that the hips are not poking out behind you.

Keep the shoulders, arms, hands, neck, and face relaxed. Be sure to keep the knees pointing over the toes for the entire exercise. Avoid the tendency to let the knees drop together or to fall to the sides as the feet point straight ahead.

### Picture This

Imagine when you jump that your feet are made of rubber that stretches away from the floor but never releases. This stretchy feeling should keep your toes pointing when you are in the air.

### Reminders

For details, see the Reminder Glossary.

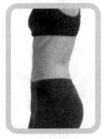 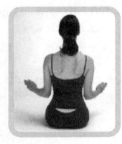 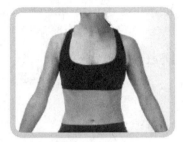

*Lifted Core*　　　　*Straight Spine*　　　　*Wide Shoulders*

# Leg Pull Back II

*For those with normal bone density only*

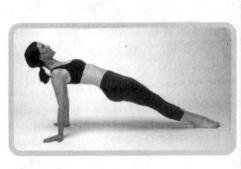 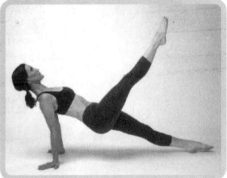

### Getting Started

With your hands slightly behind the shoulders and your legs extended out in front of you, lift your hips off of the floor. Lift the hips high enough so that you are in a straight line from head to toe.

### Moving

Lift the right leg without allowing the hips to sink. Lower the right leg and repeat with the left.

### Breathing

Exhale as you lift. Inhale as you lower.

**Repetitions:**　　3 lifts with each leg.

### Keep This in Mind

The stomach muscles need to work extra hard on this exercise to keep your hips off of the floor. Don't put all of your concentration on your legs—the abdominals will help you get the leg off the floor and to keep the hips from sagging. Push the shoulders away from the ears. Your head should be in line with the rest of your body so don't look toward your feet. Feel the spine lengthening and your head as just an extension of that line. If you find this exercise too difficult, try to just hold the "start position" then relax (in this case, repeat 6 times).

### Picture This

Imagine you are trying to keep away from a fire burning under your hips—keep lifting!

### Reminders

For details, see the Reminder Glossary.

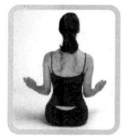
*Straight spine*

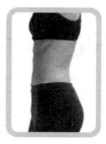
*Lifted core*

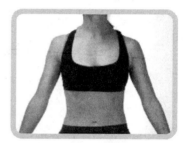
*Wide shoulders*

# Leg Pull Front II

*For those with normal bone density only*

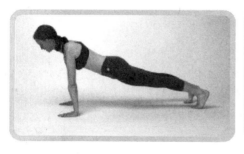
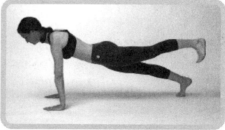

### Getting Started

Begin in plank position, lying on your stomach with your hands directly under your shoulders, legs straight and squeezing together, and toes tucked under. Straighten your arms. Now your weight should be distributed between your hands and your feet.

## Moving

Keeping the shoulders and arms still, lift the right leg without changing the shape of the spine. Now, put it back down. Repeat with the left leg.

## Breathing

Exhale, lift the leg. Inhale, bring the leg back down.

## Repetitions: 3 lifts with each leg.

## Keep This in Mind

Do not allow your spine to come out of alignment by looking up with the chin (you must keep it tucked, looking at the floor) or by allowing the hips to lift as you lift the leg. You should be in a nice long line from heels to the crown of your head. Keep the shoulders pressing away from your ears and back.

Don't shift from side to side as you alternate legs. The less you shift, the more you will be using the abdominals. It's exercises such as this that I love for the abdominals—they are working like crazy, but they are long and not crunched. That's exactly what you'll be creating, too—long abs, not crunched or poochy abs.

## Picture This

Imagine that you have a teacup resting on your hips and shoulders so that when you lift one leg off the floor you don't tilt to one side and spill the tea.

## Reminders:

For details, see Reminder Glossary.

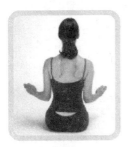
*Straight Spine*

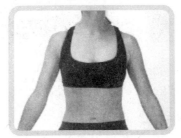
*Wide Shoulders*

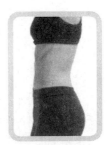
*Lifted Core*

# Neck Pull

*For those with normal bone density only*

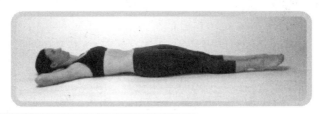

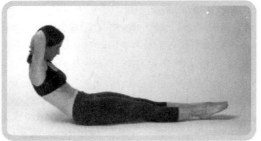

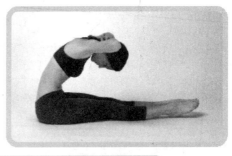

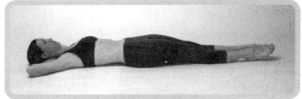

### Getting Started

Lie on your back with your hands clasped behind your head. Allow the elbows to relax open, and keep them open for the entire exercise. Legs are squeezing together. Spine is neutral (ribs are not protruding and the spine is not flat on the floor).

### Moving

Begin by tucking the chin in 1 inch without lifting the head. Now lift the head over the neck, the neck over the shoulders, the shoulders over the ribs, the ribs over the hips, and then the hips over the thighs. Now, pass through each vertebra sequentially as you lower to the floor.

**Breathing**

Exhale, roll up. Inhale, pause. Exhale, roll down. Inhale, pause.

**Repetitions:** 4–8.

**Keep This in Mind**

Do not allow the elbows to come forward of your nose. The elbows should stay pressed back so that the work comes from the abdominals, not from the arms. Keeping the elbows open will also keep your shoulders wide and open. Do not allow your stomach to pooch—the abdominals should stay flat and wide without pushing out with the effort. You are trying to create a C shape with your spine as you leave the floor and then hold that C shape as long as possible on your way back down to the floor.

If this exercise is too difficult, just roll up as high as you can for 6 repetitions. Then start from sitting up with the legs still extended out in front of you and roll down as far as you can. The little toe on both feet should be pulled back toward you to keep the soles of the feet from looking at each other.

**Picture This**

Imagine that your spine is a string of pearls. As you roll up, lift the strand of pearls slowly and gently so that one little pearl comes off the floor at a time. You can also imagine that someone is standing behind you, pulling your elbows back continuously.

**Reminders**

For details, see the Reminder Glossary.

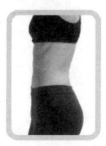
*Lifted Core*

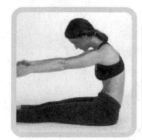
*C-shaped Spine*

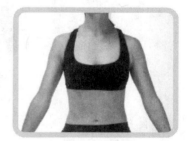
*Wide Shoulders*

# Open Leg Rocker

*For those with normal bone density only*

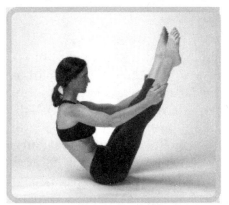

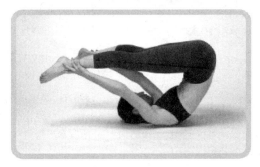

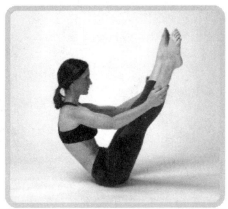

### Getting Started

Place the soles of your feet together. Hold on to your legs just below the knees and lean back as far as you can to create a C shape with your spine. Extend one leg up and only slightly out from the shoulder. Now the other leg joins. Continue to pull your stomach muscles back to keep your spine in a C shape for the entire exercise.

## Moving

Holding on to your legs, allow yourself to rock back to your shoulders and then back up to your start position. Hold the start position before you repeat the exercise.

## Breathing

Inhale, rock back. Exhale, return to start.

## Repetitions: 4–8.

## Let's Make This a Little Easier

Instead of straightening the legs, start sitting up with the knees up and soles of the feet down. Hold on just below the knees and pull your abdominals as far away from the thighs as you can, but don't hunch the shoulders. Lift your toes off the mat 1 inch and begin rocking. Don't allow the toes to touch the mat until you have performed six or eight repetitions.

## Keep This in Mind

Do not use momentum or throw your head back to get you going on this exercise. Very little momentum is involved. It is all about engaging your abdominal muscles to control the exercise. If you are doing the modified version, keep working on your flexibility. With soles of the feet together, straighten one leg and put it back down. Repeat, with the other leg. You'll be more flexible before you know it. Be sure to hold the C shape in your spine, whether you are doing the exercise or its modified version.

## Picture This

Imagine that you are 4 years old again and that you just got a brand-new rocking horse for your birthday. Smoothly rock back and forth as if you were suspended by springs.

## Reminders

For details, see the Reminder Glossary.

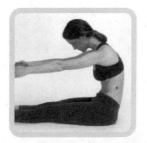
*C-shaped Spine*

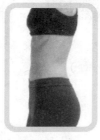
*Lifted Core*

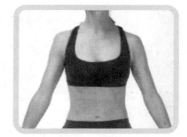
*Wide Shoulders*

# Push-Ups

*For those with normal bone density only*

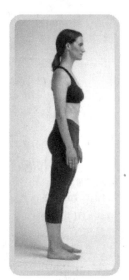
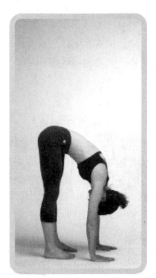

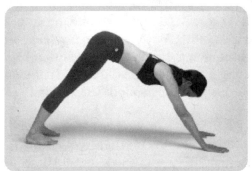

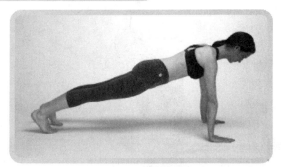

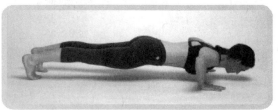

### Getting Started

Start by standing in perfect alignment (see Chapter 3). Look straight ahead, with shoulders wide, arms relaxed, and feet about hip-distance apart and pointing straight ahead.

### Moving

Drop your chin to your neck and roll down your spine one vertebra at a time. Once your hands are on the floor (you can bend your knees if you need to), walk your hands out in front of you. Keep walking forward until you are in a plank position with the toes tucked under and shoulders over the hands. From this position, bend your elbows as much as you can and then straighten them again. Now, walk yourself back in towards your feet and roll sequentially up the spine, back to your perfectly aligned starting position.

### Breathing

Exhale, roll down. Inhale, walk out to a plank position. Exhale, bend the elbows. Inhale, straighten the elbows. Exhale, walk your self back in. Inhale, roll up.

### Repetitions:  3–5.

### Keep This in Mind

Pay special attention to your alignment at the start position. If you need more posture guidelines, see *Golden Rule #5* in Chapter 3 (page 65). When you reach your plank position, make sure your hips are not still sticking up. If your hips are not sticking up, you should be able to place a plank from your head to your heels. The plank should be touching the back of your head, shoulders, hips, and heels, if you are perfectly aligned. When you lower your elbows, keep your chin tucked and be sure to bring the hips down with you—don't hike them up as you lower the shoulders.

### Picture This

When creating the plank position to perform the actual push-up, imagine that you are "light as a feather and stiff as a board." Remember that game?

### Reminders

For details, see the Reminder Glossary.

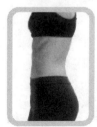 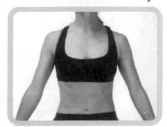 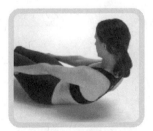

*Lifted Core*          *Wide Shoulders*          *Work Sequentially*

# Rollover

*For those with normal bone density only*

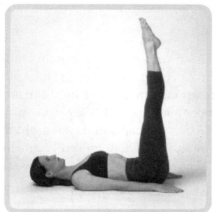

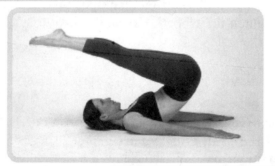

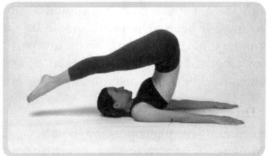

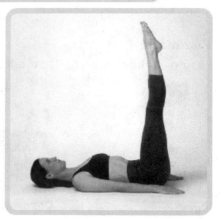

### Getting Started

Lie on your back with your feet pointed to the ceiling and hip-width apart. Keep the shoulders wide and pressed into the floor. Reach your fingers long past your hips to help bring the shoulders away from the ears.

### Moving

Pull the lowest abdominal muscles (the ones about 4 inches below your navel) down to the spine. This small movement will initiate the *Rollover*. Press into the floor with the backs of your arms as you continue to squeeze the abdominals to the spine in order to take the legs overhead. Once overhead, bring the legs together and roll back down, keeping the legs together. Return to your start position.

### Breathing

Exhale, roll over. Inhale, bring the legs together. Exhale, roll down. Inhale, take the legs to hip-width apart.

### Repetitions: 3–6.

### Keep This in Mind

Do not initiate this exercise with a swinging motion of the legs—be sure to use the abdominals and arms instead. There is a tendency to allow the chin to jut toward the ceiling, so keep the chin tucked and the back of the neck reaching toward the floor. Keep the legs straight and strong. Keep the soles of the feet from looking at each other by pulling back the little toes on both feet.

### Picture This

Imagine that the pressure you are putting on the backs of your arms is exerting a force on an imaginary pump under your hips. The harder you press your arms, the higher the pump lifts your hips.

### Reminders

For details, see the Reminder Glossary.

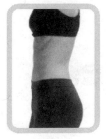 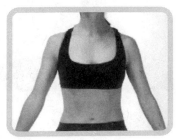 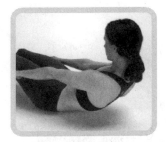

*Lifted Core*      *Wide Shoulders*      *Work Sequentially*

# Roll-Up

*For those with normal bone density only*

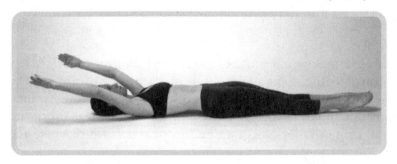

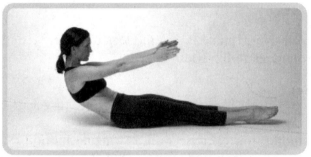

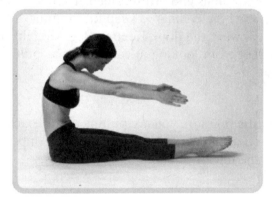

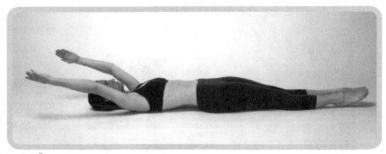

## Getting Started

Lie on your back with your legs together and flat on the floor. Keep every single vertebra flat on the mat as you carry your arms overhead. Do not allow the spine to release from the mat in your start position.

## Moving

Bring your arms over your shoulders and create a C shape with your spine by doing the following: Tuck your chin 1 inch without lifting the head. Now, bring your head over your neck, neck over your shoulders, shoulders over your ribs, ribs over your hips, and finally your hips over your thighs. Pause for a moment before you roll back down. Once down, take your arms back overhead without releasing the spine from the floor.

## Breathing

Exhale, roll up. Inhale, pause. Exhale, roll down. Inhale, pause.

## Repetitions:  5–8.

## Keep This in Mind

Stay relaxed and do not allow tension to build up, especially in the shoulder and neck region. Keep stretching your legs long, and that will help to keep them from peeling away from the mat as you roll up.

Keep the legs together and you will be working the inner thighs as well as the abdominal muscles. Keep the little toes pulled back toward you to keep the bottoms of the feet from looking at each other and to keep the feet properly aligned.

Keep this exercise smooth. Do not "jerk" through the roll-up—if you can't get up all the way without jerking through the middle, then only go up as high as you can. Then start sitting up and roll down as far as you can without "dropping" down to the floor.

## Picture This

Imagine that a large ball is resting on your stomach. When you roll up, don't crush the ball. Instead, imagine arcing over it.

## Reminders

For details, see the Reminder Glossary.

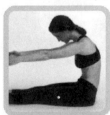
*C-shaped Spine*

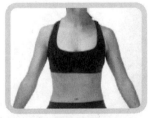
*Wide Shoulders*

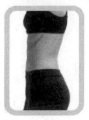
*Lifted Core*

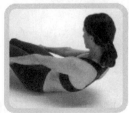
*Work Sequentially*

# The Saw

*For those with normal bone density only*

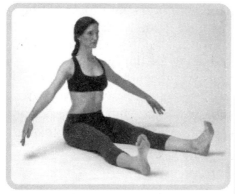

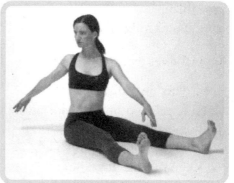

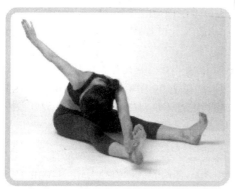

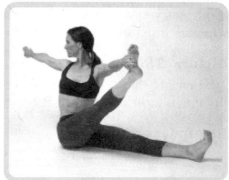

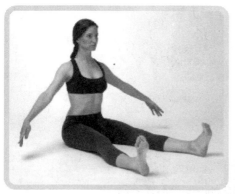

### Getting Started

Sit up straight with your legs extended in front of you about shoulder-width apart. If you can't sit up straight with the legs extended, find a phone book or a few firm pillows to sit on. Extend your arms out to your sides.

### Moving

Twist the shoulders (the arms only go along for the ride) toward your right foot. Now look at your right hand as you reach for the little toe of your right foot with your left pinky finger. If you can reach the toe, then grab the outside of the foot and lift. Continue twisting and looking behind yourself. Come back up to the twisted position and then return to your start position. Repeat on the left.

### Breathing

Exhale as you twist. Continue the same exhale as you "saw." Inhale, return to the twist, and return to start.

### Repetitions:  4–8.

### Let's Make This a Little Easier

If you can't reach your little toe, just leave out the part where you lift the leg off of the floor.

### Keep This in Mind

*The Saw* should be a gentle twisting motion. Do not force the twist or jerk quickly into the twist. This is a gentle stretch for the spine and the backs of the legs, so be gentle with yourself.

To intensify the stretch, pull the little toe back toward you on each leg. Do not allow the soles of the feet to look at each other. Twisting motions of the spine allow the lungs to be completely "wrung out" of air. So be sure to exhale as you twist, not inhale.

### Picture This

Imagine that you are sawing off the little toe with the pinky finger.

### Reminders

For details, see the Reminder Glossary.

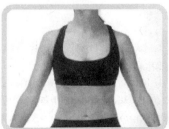
*Wide Shoulders*

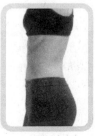
*Lifted Core*

# Side Kicks V: Hip Hinges

*For those with normal bone density only*

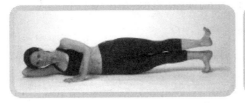
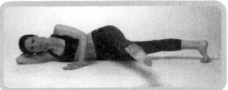
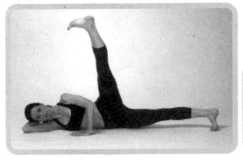
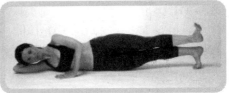

## Getting Started

Lie on your right side with hip over hip and shoulder over shoulder. Your right leg should be turned out so that you are "standing" on the right toes with the leg straight and the knee pulled off of the mat for the entire exercise. Start with your left leg resting on your right, with the left foot pointing forward. Lift your waist off the mat.

## Moving

Carry the left leg forward as far as it can comfortably go. Now turn the toes of the left leg up to face the ceiling. Carry the left leg up so it is not quite over the hip. Now lower the left heel to touch the right heel. Return the left foot to its start position.

## Breathing

Exhale, carry the leg forward. Inhale, turn the toes to face the ceiling. Exhale, carry the leg up. Inhale, lower the leg.

## Repetitions: 8.

## Keep This in Mind

The hips and shoulders should not rock back and forth while you perform *Side Kicks V*. This is tough, but you can do it. Isolate all of the movement at the hip joint only. I recommend lining yourself up against a wall so that you can just barely feel the wall on your back. As you perform the exercise, you shouldn't feel any more or any less pressure from the wall. Be sure not to allow the "standing" leg to bend or the waist to drop onto the mat. Keep lengthening actively through the top of the head and in the opposite direction with the heel of the "standing" leg. This is a very active exercise for every part of the body. Don't allow your upper body to relax.

### Picture This

Imagine that your hip is a doorknob that is being turned. The turning motion opens the "door" as your leg lifts over your hip.

### Reminders

For details, see the Reminder Glossary.

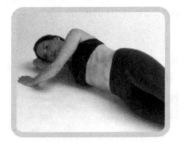 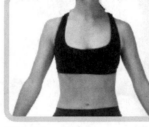 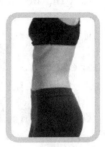

*Hip Over Hip...*          *Wide Shoulders*          *Lifted Core*

## Side Kicks VI: Beats

*For those with normal bone density only*

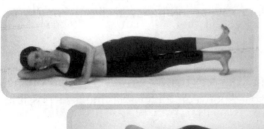

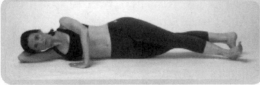

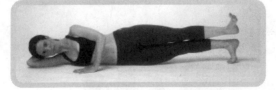

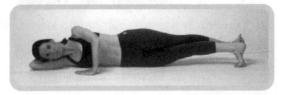

### Getting Started

Lie on your right side with hip over hip and shoulder over shoulder. Your bottom leg should be turned out so that you are "standing" on the toes with the leg straight and knee pulled off of the mat for the entire exercise. The top leg is resting on the bottom with the foot flexed and toes pointing toward the ceiling. Your waist is lifted.

### Moving

Raise the left leg as high as your flexibility will allow, and bring the heel of the flexed foot onto the floor directly in front of the right leg. Raise the left leg again and bring the heel down again to touch the floor behind the right leg.

### Breathing

Inhale, lift. Exhale, lower.

### Repetitions: 8.

### Keep This in Mind

These are quick beats, but you must maintain control of your legs. Do not throw your leg up with abandon and then allow it to collapse back down. Keep your core lifted and do not roll back as the leg kicks upward. Most people do not have the range of motion to get the working leg to point directly to the ceiling when lifted. Have the working leg come slightly in front of you as you kick in order to avoid rolling, even slightly, onto your back.

### Picture This

Imagine that you are squeezing your legs between two very narrow panes of glass. You want to narrow the space between the glass as much as possible.

### Reminders

For details, see the Reminder Glossary.

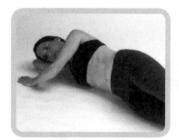
*Hip Over Hip...*

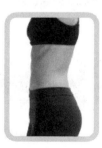
*Lifted Core*

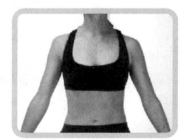
*Wide Shoulders*

# Single Leg Stretch II

*For those with normal bone density only*

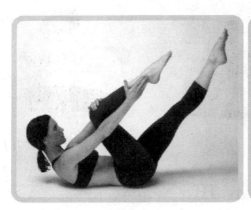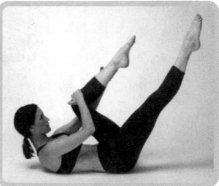

### Getting Started

Lie on your back with the left leg extended to about 45 degrees from the floor and the right leg bent. Hold the right knee with the left hand and the right ankle with the right hand. (When you change legs, remember that the outside hand always goes to the ankle). Lift your head and shoulders off the mat.

### Moving

Change legs so that the left leg bends and the right leg extends.

### Breathing

Exhale for two changes. Inhale for two changes.

### Repetitions: 8–16 changes.

### Keep This in Mind

Keep the bent leg aligned and straight, not turned out. You can achieve this by pushing into the outside hand with the ankle. Maintain a circle of tension from the arms, through the shoulders, down the spine, and back up the bent knee. This is easily achieved by pulling the abdominal muscles flat while gently pushing away and into the hand with the knee that is bent. Keep the chin gently tucked.

### Picture This

Imagine a mass of energy that circles from the chest, through the arms, down the thigh of the bent leg, up the stomach, and back to the chest. This energy is vibrating and keeping the thigh as far away from the chest as possible.

### Reminders

For details, see the Reminder Glossary.

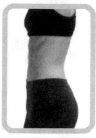
*Lifted Core*

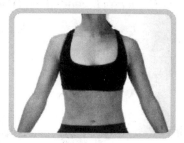
*Wide Shoulders*

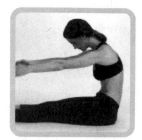
*C-shaped Spine*

# Swan III

*For those with normal bone density only*

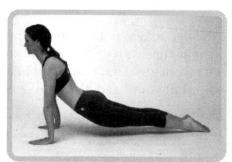

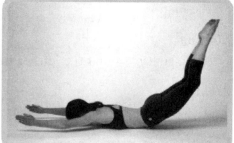

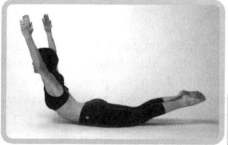

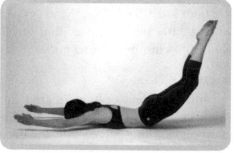

### Getting Started

This is an advanced exercise. Lie on your stomach with your hands directly under your shoulders. Legs are stretched long and hip-width apart. Straighten your arms and allow your hipbones to leave the floor, but be sure to keep the abdominal muscles pulled toward your spine. Press your shoulders down.

### Moving

Throw your arms out in front of you and allow the legs to kick into the air. As the legs lower, allow the arms to rock back up. After two rocks, catch yourself back in the start position.

### Breathing

Exhale as you toss the arms. Inhale as you toss the legs.

### Repetitions:    2–6.

### Keep This in Mind

This exercise should rock back and forth with fluidity. Imagine that your limbs are being stretched away from your center, while pushing your shoulder blades toward your hips. When the spine is extended, there is actually more space between the vertebrae. Try to feel this space while you perform *Swan III,* and that will keep you from feeling crunched. Keep the chin gently tucked so that your head is an extension of the spine, not a break backwards.

### Picture This

Imagine when you begin this exercise that you have a ball resting on your feet. After you drop the arms out from under you, vigorously toss the ball from your feet to your hands. Now throw the arms up with a lot of energy in order to get the ball back to the feet.

### Reminders

For details, see the Reminder Glossary.

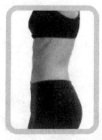
*Lifted Core*

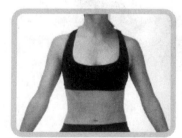
*Wide Shoulders*

# Teaser I

*For those with normal bone density only*

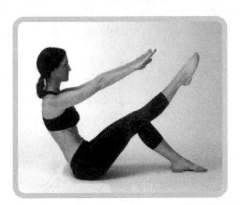

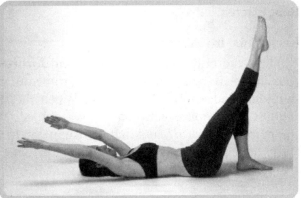

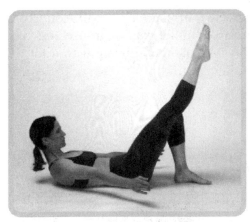

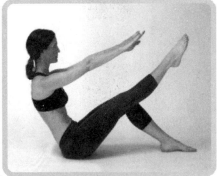

### Getting Started

Sit up straight with knees up and soles of the feet on the floor. Hold onto your knees with both hands and pull the stomach away from the thighs. Now maintain that shape while you point one foot up to the ceiling and point the hands up to the lifted foot.

### Moving

While maintaining the rounded shape of the lower spine, roll down until you feel your low back touch the floor. Continue to roll down vertebra by vertebra. Once lowered, take the arms overhead. Swing your arms wide out to your sides and then down to your hips. Now, roll back up to your start position.

### Breathing

Exhale, roll down. Inhale, pause. Exhale, roll up. Inhale, pause.

**Repetitions:**  4 sets of 2 complete breaths.

### Keep This in Mind

This is an abdominal exercise that concentrates on length, not crunching. Your arms are long, your legs are long, and even your spine is long as you roll up and down. Be sure to feel your low back roll down to the floor one vertebra at a time. Don't "clunk" down onto the floor with a flat back.

Keep your shoulders wide and open by gently pinching the shoulder blades together. Don't allow your shoulders to round even though the spine is rounded. The spine is not connected to the shoulders, so just because the back is rounding doesn't mean the shoulders must also.

### Picture This

Imagine that the lifted leg is attached to a rope that is attached to the wall in front of you. The rope continuously pulls and keeps the leg in a stretched position.

### Reminders

For details, see the Reminder Glossary.

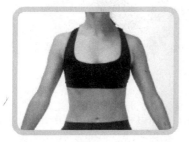
*Wide Shoulders*

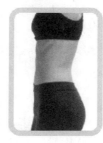
*Lifted Core*

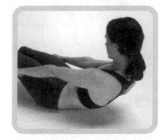
*Work Sequentially*

# Teaser II

*For those with normal bone density only*

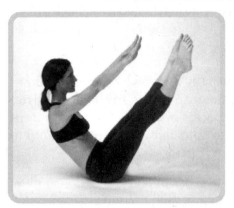

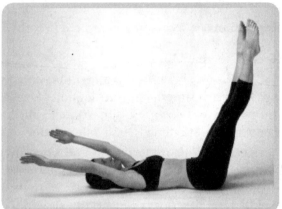

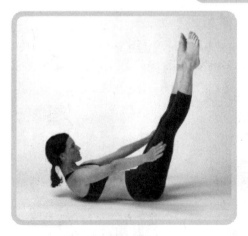

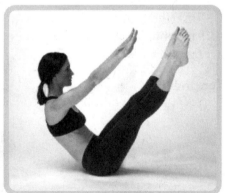

## Getting Started

Sitting with the soles of the feet together and hands on the lower legs, lean back in order to pull the stomach into the spine and away from the thighs. Now, straighten one leg up and in front of your shoulder, and then the other. Let go of the legs and point the hands up and past the feet.

## Moving

Keep the legs where they are and roll down the spine until you feel the mid-back on the floor. The arms go overhead and then swing wide to the sides of your body. As the arms come back toward the hips, roll back up the spine, vertebra by vertebra, until you are back in your start position.

## Breathing

Exhale, roll down. Inhale, arms go overhead. Exhale, roll back up. Inhale, pause.

## Repetitions:  2–4.

## Keep This in Mind

This exercise is tough! Do not overdo it. If you do too many and allow your stomach to "pooch," you will be building bulky stomach muscles instead of long, lean muscles. For that reason, be sure to keep the abdominal muscles pulled tight to your spine—especially the lowest 4 inches of the abdominals.

As the arms go overhead, keep every vertebra in contact with the floor. Keep the legs lengthening toward the ceiling and the arms reaching long away from the center of your body.

## Picture This

Imagine that your legs are resting in straps that are hanging from the ceiling. Once you are flat on the floor with your arms overhead, imagine that you are making an angel in the snow by swinging your arms as wide as possible out to your sides and down to your hips as your roll back up to your start position.

## Reminders

For details, see the Reminder Glossary.

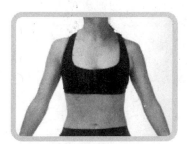 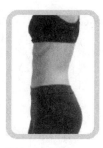 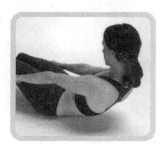

*Wide Shoulders*          *Lifted Core*          *Work Sequentially*

# Teaser III

*For those with normal bone density only*

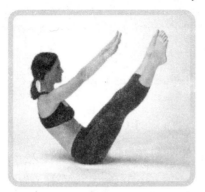

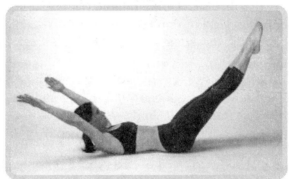

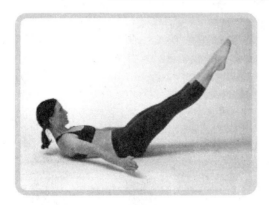

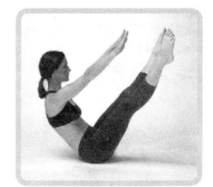

### Getting Started

Sitting with the soles of the feet together and hands on the lower leg, lean back in order to pull the stomach into the spine and away from the thighs. Now, straighten one leg up and in front of your shoulder, and then the other. Let go of the legs and point the hands up and past the feet.

## Moving

Roll down sequentially to your mid-back as you lower the legs toward the floor at the same time. Now, take the arms overhead and circle them wide and back around to point at the feet. As the arms circle, begin rolling up through the spine and bring the legs back to their start position.

## Breathing

Exhale, roll down. Inhale, arms go overhead. Exhale, roll back up. Inhale, pause.

## Repetitions:  2–4.

## Keep This in Mind

This is the toughest of all the *Teasers*—go easy. This exercise is about length, so be careful that you don't feel crunched and curled. The only part of your body that should be curling is your low to mid-back. Everything else is stretched long. The toes are pointing and the fingers are reaching.

As you open the arms and legs toward the floor, imagine that your toes and fingers are connected by a rubber band so that the limbs will lower gently and with a little resistance. In other words, don't allow the limbs to flop open.

Be careful that you don't go so low with the legs that the stomach pooches or that the spine pulls even one millimeter away from the mat. You will find that your legs will probably not go quite as low if you keep your spine and stomach still. That's good! You will be building much, much flatter abdominals if you keep within your range.

## Picture This

Imagine that this is an easy exercise...feel better now? Imagine that your arms and legs are attached by a rubber band. Feel the tension connecting your limbs and gently stretch the band apart as you lower.

## Reminders

For details, see the Reminder Glossary.

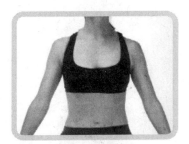
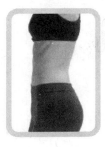
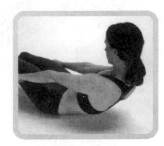

*Wide Shoulders*            *Lifted Core*            *Work Sequentially*

# Twist

*For those with normal bone density only*

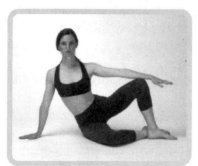

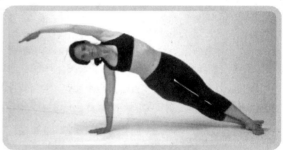

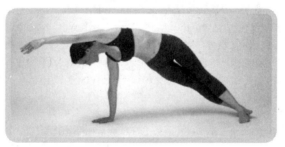

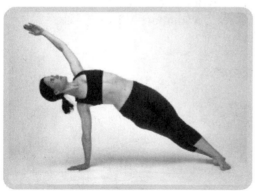

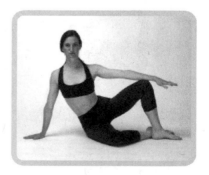

### Getting Started

Sit on your right hip with your right hand on the floor slightly away from your shoulder. Your left hand is resting on your left knee. Your legs are slightly bent with the sole of the left foot on the floor in front of the right foot.

### Moving

Lift your hips off the floor as your straighten both legs. Your right shoulder should come directly over your right hand as the legs straighten and push you in that direction. Once lifted, keep the right shoulder still and twist to look at the floor. Now twist to look at the ceiling. Come back to center and return to your start position.

### Breathing

Inhale, lift. Exhale, twist to the floor. Inhale, twist back to center. Exhale, twist to the ceiling. Inhale, twist back to center. Exhale, return to sitting.

### Repetitions:   1–3.

### Keep This in Mind

This is a very advanced exercise. If you are having trouble, try doing only the first part. Lift the hips and immediately come back down without twisting. This exercise emphasizes shoulder stability, abdominal control, stretching, and lengthening.

Don't allow the working shoulder to relax and push up to your ear. Actively keep the abdominals pulled in and up. In order to get the hips off the floor, push through the sole of the foot of the top leg. Keep length in your body by imagining the toes and fingers pulling away from each other in the longest possible arc that passes through the ribs that aface the ceiling.

### Picture This

Once you are lifted, imagine that your supporting arm and shoulder is a fulcrum around which you are rotating the rest of your body, as you look toward the floor and then toward the ceiling.

### Reminders

For details, see the Reminder Glossary.

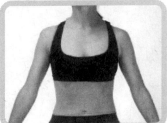
*Wide Shoulders*

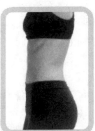
*Lifted Core*

# OsteoPilates Programs for Those With Normal Bone Density Only

These exercise programs are designed for total fitness. The programs that are created here combine exercises from both indexes of exercises in this book—for normal bone density and for osteoporosis. The exercises that are safe specifically for those with osteoporosis or osteopoenia are real Pilates exercises that simply don't create a fracture-risk situation for those individuals with low bone density. When you come across an exercise that is in the osteoporosis program, do not skip it thinking that it will be too easy. They vary in difficulty, just as the exercises in the index for normal bone density do. All of the exercises listed in these programs are important for complete and balanced strength and flexibility. To indicate where you can look to find more information about a specific exercise, I have placed an *L* after the exercises that are in the previous chapter for those with low bone density. The rest can be found in this chapter, for those with normal bone density. Enjoy!

## Beginning Program for Normal Bone Density

**Breathing** —*L*     **Toe Touches** —*L*     **Bridging** —*L*

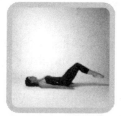
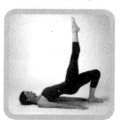

*Page 123*     *Page 173*     *Page 125*

**The Hundred II**     **Low Back Stretch** —*L*     **Single Leg Stretch II**

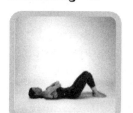
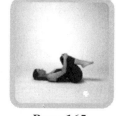
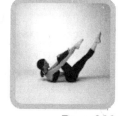

*Page 187*     *Page 165*     *Page 209*

**Teaser I**     **Roll-Up**     **The Saw**

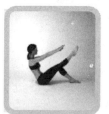
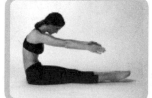
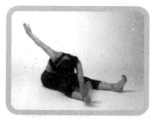

*Page 212*     *Page 202*     *Page 204*

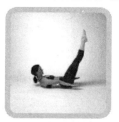
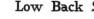
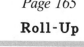

### Puppet —L

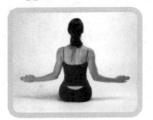

Page 129

### Side Kicks I —L

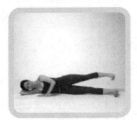

Page 153

### Side Kicks II —L

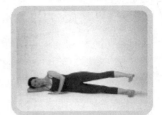

Page 155

### Side Kicks III —L

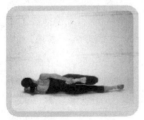

Page 157

### Side Kicks IV —L

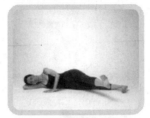

Page 159

### Hamstring Stretch —L

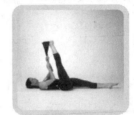

Page 165

### Quadricep Stretch —L

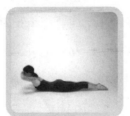

Page 166

### Swan I —L

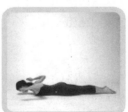

Page 167

### Swan II —L

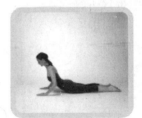

Page 169

### Single Leg Kick —L

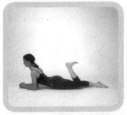

Page 161

### Elbow Lifts —L

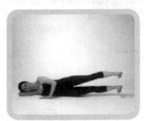

Page 137

### Leg Pull Front II

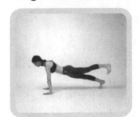

Page 192

**Balance—*L***

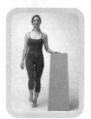

*Page 121*

**Push-Ups**

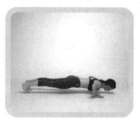

*Page 198*

**Shoulder Stretch—*L***

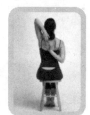

*Page 149*

# Intermediate Program for Normal Bone Density

**Breathing—*L***

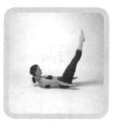

*Page 123*

**Toe Touches—*L***

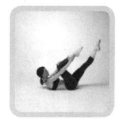

*Page 173*

**Bridging—*L***

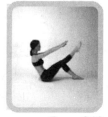

*Page 125*

**The Hundred II**

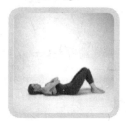

*Page 187*

**Single Leg Stretch II**

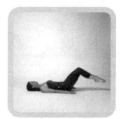

*Page 209*

**Teaser I**

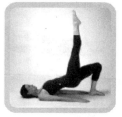

*Page 212*

**Teaser II**

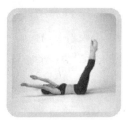

*Page 214*

**Rollover**

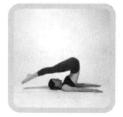

*Page 200*

**Roll-up**

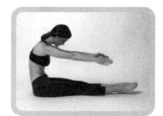

*Page 202*

### Open Leg Rocker

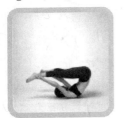

*Page 196*

### The Saw

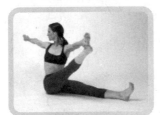

*Page 204*

### Mermaid —*L*

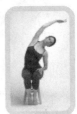

*Page 145*

### Side Kicks I —*L*

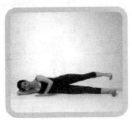

*Page 153*

### Side Kicks II —*L*

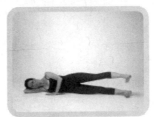

*Page 155*

### Side Kicks III —*L*

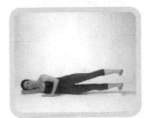

*Page 157*

### Side Kicks V

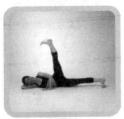

*Page 206*

### Hamstring Stretch —*L*

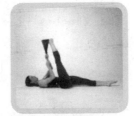

*Page 165*

### Quadricep Stretch —*L*

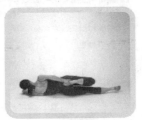

*Page 166*

### Swan I —*L*

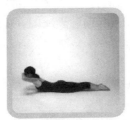

*Page 167*

### Swan II —*L*

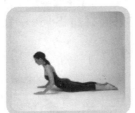

*Page 169*

### Elbow Lifts —*L*

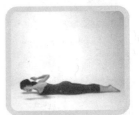

*Page 137*

### Double Leg Kick —L

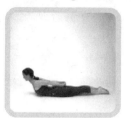

*Page 133*

### Swimming —L

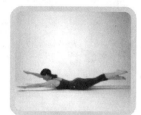

*Page 171*

### Leg Pull Front II

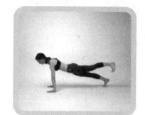

*Page 192*

### Leg Pull Back II

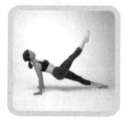

*Page 191*

### Push-Ups

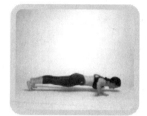

*Page 198*

### Jumping

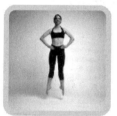

*Page 190*

## Advanced Program for Normal Bone Density

### Breathing —L

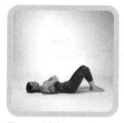

*Page 123*

### Toe Touches —L

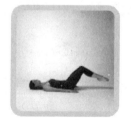

*Page 173*

### The Hundred II

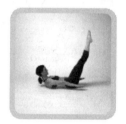

*Page 187*

### Bridging

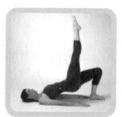

*Page 125*

### Single Leg Stretch II

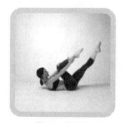

*Page209*

### Double Leg Stretch II

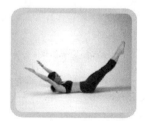

*Page 185*

**Corkscrew**

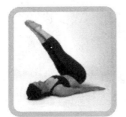

*Page 183*

**Jackknife**

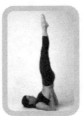

*Page 188*

**Teaser III**

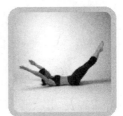

*Page 216*

**Neck Pull**

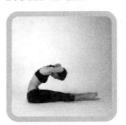

*Page 194*

**Open Leg Rocker**

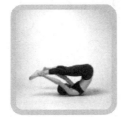

*Page 196*

**The Saw**

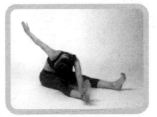

*Page 204*

**Puppet —L**

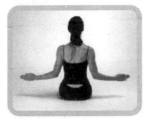

*Page 129*

**Side Kicks I —L**

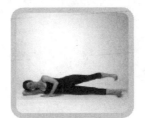

*Page 153*

**Side Kicks II —L**

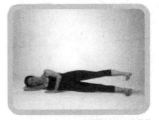

*Page 155*

**Side Kicks III —L**

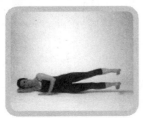

*Page 157*

**Side Kicks V**

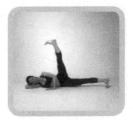

*Page 206*

**Side Kicks VI**

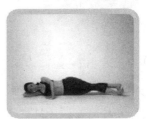

*Page 207*

### Hamstring Stretch—L
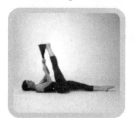
Page 165

### Quadricep Stretch—L
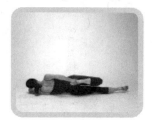
Page 166

### Swan I—L
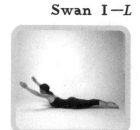
Page 167

### Swan II—L
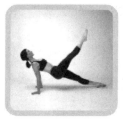
Page 169

### Swan III
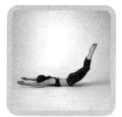
Page 210

### Leg Pull Front II
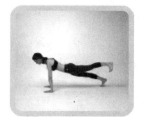
Page 192

### Leg Pull Back II
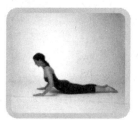
Page 191

### Twist
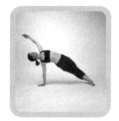
Page 218

### Push-Ups
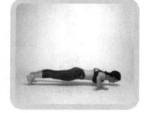
Page 198

### Jumping
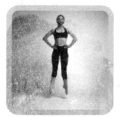
Page 190

### Shoulder Stretch—L
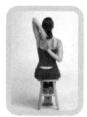
Page 149

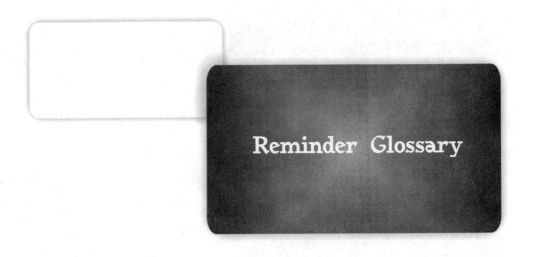

# Reminder Glossary

## Work Sequentially

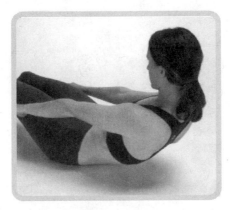

In an abdominal exercise where you have to roll through the spine, be sure to allow time for each vertebra to hit individually. Most people have a section of the spine that doesn't want to "roll through" an exercise. Slow down and give it time to work. You can also imagine your spine as a pearl necklace, where each little pearl is lowered or lifted separately.

## C-shaped Spine

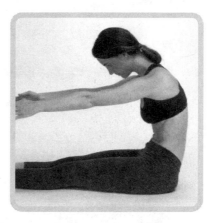

To achieve a C-shaped spine, imagine an arc from your head to your tailbone. Don't over-curve. Imagine that you are arcing over a giant ball and that you don't want to squeeze the ball flat.

# Wide Shoulders

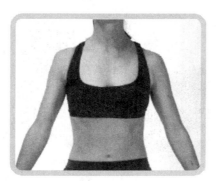

To find the perfect spot for your shoulders, extend both arms out to your sides. Now lower your arms, imagining that your shoulders are still out where your fingertips were. Using this technique will prevent rounded shoulders during all of the exercises.

# Lifted Core

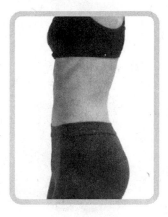

The core muscles will be working during every exercise if you always keep the stomach muscles lifted toward the spine and up and under the ribcage. Be sure not to lift the shoulders when you lift the abdominals. This lift is possible, not only with all of the exercises, but all day, everyday. You'll be amazed at the improvement in your stomach muscles because of this simple exercise.

# Flat Spine

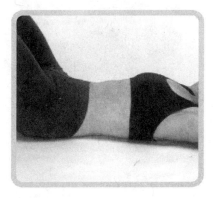

During some exercises, in order to keep the abdominals working correctly, the spine must be pressed flat into the floor. Do not allow it to peel away even a *millimeter* while performing the exercises. Work correctly and you will get the results you are seeking.

# Straight Spine

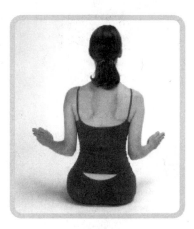

A straight spine is actually a neutral spine. If you were to back up against a wall, your head, shoulders, and hips should touch the wall. The back of your neck and your low back should be slightly curved away from the wall.

# Hip Over Hip and Shoulder Over Shoulder

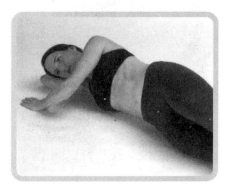

It is very easy to allow the hips and shoulders to roll around. Keep them very, very still in order to make the legs and core work correctly.

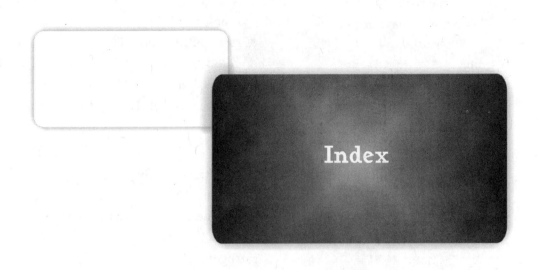

# Index

hot flashes, 40
  soy for reduced, 51
hundred I, the, 139-141
hundred II, the, 187-188
hypercalciuria, 23
hyperparathyroidism, 20
hypertension, 21
hypogonadism, 20

## I

IBD, 21
illnesses and their treatments, 26
immobility, 22
inactive lifestyle, 22
inflammatory bowel disease, 21
insomnia, 41

## J

jackknife, 188-189
jumping, 190-191

## K

kick, double leg, 133-135
kick, single leg, 161-163
kicks I, side, front/back,
  153-155
kicks II, side, small circles,
  155-157
kicks III, side, lower leg lift,
  157-159
kicks IV, side, rotations,
  159-161
kicks V, side, hip hinges,
  206-207
kicks VI, side, beats, 207-208

## L

lactose intolerance, 77
leg kick, double, 133-135
leg pull back I, 141-142
leg pull back II, 191-192
leg pull front I, 143-145
leg pull front II, 192-193
leg rocker, open, 196-197
leg stretch, double, 135-137
leg stretch I, single,
  163-165
leg stretch II, double,
  185-186
leg stretch II, single,
  209-210
legs, do not abduct your, 62
libido, 41
list of understanding, 72
lupus, 22

## M

medicine, complementary, 48-50
memory, 42
menopausal symptoms,
  botanical treatments of,
    46-47
  temporary, 52
menopause by ethnicity, 50
menopause, 20, 37, 38, 43
  African-American, 50-51
  Asian, 51
  Caucasian, 51
  Hispanic, 50
menstrual cycle, irregular, 40
mermaid, 145-147
motivation, 103

# About the Author

KARENA LINEBACK comes to Pilates from a professional dance career. Dancers have been using Pilates for more than 70 years to maintain long, lean physiques while tremendously increasing their strength. It wasn't a big leap then, when she retired from dancing to open her own Pilates studio.

Karena's interest in tailoring exercise programs to fit very individual needs directed her to become certified in Pilates post-rehabilitation by Polestar Education. She also holds certifications from the PhysicalMind Institute, as well as the American Council on Exercise. Her study of kinesiology and anatomy at the University of Utah are a part of her ongoing study of movement.

Karena's vast teaching experience in her own studio, several dozen dance studios around the nation and at the College of the Canyons (Santa Clarita, California), Salisbury State University (Salisbury, Maryland), and as a guest teacher at George Washington University (Washington D.C.) make her a master Pilates teacher. She has dedicated her professional life to understanding the human body and to improving the lives of hundreds of people who participate in her Pilates programs.

Karena lives in Santa Clarita, California with her husband and son. She can be reached at Karena@osteopilates.com.